GREAT
SEX
FOR
HARD
TIMES

GREAT SEX

FOR HARD TIMES

KIM SWITNICKI

BERKLEY BOOKS, NEW YORK

THE BERKLEY PUBLISHING GROUP
Published by the Penguin Group
Penguin Group (USA) Inc.
375 Hudson Street, New York, New York 10014, USA
Penguin Group (Canada), 90 Eglinton Avenue East, Suite 700, Toronto, Ontario M4P 2Y3, Canada
(a division of Pearson Penguin Canada Inc.)
Penguin Books Ltd., 80 Strand, London WC2R 0RL, England
Penguin Group Ireland, 25 St. Stephen's Green, Dublin 2, Ireland (a division of Penguin Books Ltd.)
Penguin Group (Australia), 250 Camberwell Road, Camberwell, Victoria 3124, Australia
(a division of Pearson Australia Group Pty. Ltd.)
Penguin Books India Pvt. Ltd., 11 Community Centre, Panchsheel Park, New Delhi—110 017, India
Penguin Group (NZ), 67 Apollo Drive, Rosedale, North Shore, 0632, New Zealand
(a division of Pearson New Zealand Ltd.)
Penguin Books (South Africa) (Pty.) Ltd., 24 Sturdee Avenue, Rosebank, Johannesburg 2196,
South Africa

Penguin Books Ltd., Registered Offices: 80 Strand, London WC2R 0RL, England

The publisher does not have any control over and does not assume any responsibility for author or third-party websites or their content. Every effort has been made to ensure that the information contained in this book is complete and accurate. However, neither the publisher nor the author is engaged in rendering professional advice or services to the individual reader. The ideas, procedures, and suggestions contained in this book are not intended as a substitute for consulting with your physician. All matters regarding your health require medical supervision. Neither the author nor the publisher shall be liable or responsible for any loss or damage allegedly arising from any information or suggestion in this book.

Copyright © 2010 Kim Switnicki
Interior illustration credits are listed on page 265.
Cover design by Erika Fusari
Cover photograph © Tony Rusecki/Alamy
Book design by Joanna Williams

BERKLEY® is a registered trademark of Penguin Group (USA) Inc.
The "B" design is a trademark of Penguin Group (USA) Inc.

PRINTING HISTORY
Berkley trade paperback edition / January 2010

Library of Congress Cataloging-in-Publication Data

Switnicki, Kim.
Great sex for hard times / Kim Switnicki.
    p.   cm.

ISBN 978-0-425-23280-4
  1. Sexual intercourse.   2. Sex instruction.   I. Title.
HQ31.S995 2010
613.9'6—dc22   2009034937

PRINTED IN THE UNITED STATES OF AMERICA

10   9   8   7   6   5   4   3   2   1

For the thousands of women who have opened their hearts, poured

out their stories, and were willing to take the next step toward

making their own authentic connection.

acknowledgments

Now I understand why authors' acknowledgments can be so long. It takes so many people doing so many things to culminate in a work such as this. I also understand that not everyone, or maybe hardly anyone, will read the thank-you pages unless there's a chance that they know someone on them or they may be included themselves. If I've forgotten to include you, my sincerest apologies and a hearty thank-you!

I'd like to thank my friend, Amanda Mitchell, whose authenticity is refreshing. Her sound counsel and outrageous sense of humor kept me in line and on the path. Kim Hamer, my friend who gave her opinion and more whenever I asked, and for that I am grateful. Shawn Driscoll (super coach), who offered insights and prodding to help me see the good things happening, and the ladies in our "group" who let me focus on the book and not on what we were "supposed" to be doing. My dear friend Tammy Plett (Rev), whose contributions are longstanding and are cherished and whose artwork adds flavor to the book.

My colleague and friend Dr. Trina Read, for supporting and cheerleading me with excitement, answers, and great ideas. My friend and colleague Emaya Elfi Dillon, who continues to amaze me with her dedication to sexual healing for the planet. My colleague Rebecca Rosenblat (aka Dr. Date), who supported me before ever meeting me.

My support team—Melissa Jones and Heidi Danos, who assisted me virtually; Krista Garren, my Web mistress; Liz Taylor, my bookkeeper; and Tara Lenz, my personal assistant—who all helped keep the show rolling along smoothly, leaving me time to focus on writing, researching, and creating.

Richard Hyams and Rae Chois, my two coaches, who kept me in tune mentally and striving to do the very best I could. Thank you both for your talent and your friendship.

My masseuse, Janice Horsnell, and my chiropractor, Barry Whyte, who worked on the kinks in my shoulders, neck, and back so I could continue to work.

Kathy at BMS Enterprises, the graphics department at Sexy Living, and Kumiko at Primal Communications, for being so accommodating for my images. Robert Reinish, creator of the Kama Sutra game, for being generous with his time and photos. Adrienne Benedicks of Erotica Readers and Writers, for allowing the link to their great sexy music list.

The team at Berkley, whom I'm sure I don't know the half of, especially my editor, Andie Avila, whose questions, comments, and suggestions sculpted the book so the ideas flowed and made sense. To Andy Ball, the copyeditor, whose sharpness and eagle eye fine-tuned and zeroed in on exactly what I meant to say. And to Pam Barricklow and Tiffany Estreicher, who have done a lot of work on this book and ensured we made all our deadlines.

Colleagues from the Laguna Beach retreat, Ryan Angelo, and Lani and Allen Voivod, who helped keep me seeing the bigger picture. Wayne Kelly, who helped me feel comfortable with my radio words. Many thanks to my agent, Jessica Faust, who always shoots straight from the hip and whose experience and manner I count on being with me for every aspect of this exciting journey.

The "boys" at Kayla's birthday party who openly shared with me their thoughts on oral sex while their sweethearts ate, swam, and played.

My sister and brother, who accepted my working on my manuscript while I was with them for a first-time-in-twenty-years-together holiday. My mom, Joan Hill, for instilling in me the survivor spirit to do what I do every day. My dad, George Stokes, who keeps waiting to see me on *Oprah* and keeps calling me the new Dr. Ruth. My father, Glen May, who may finally give up the thought that I should get a job.

Dr. Ruth and Canada's own version, Sue Johanson, who paved the way for women like me to help women like you. All the other wonderful sex experts and writers whose work has increased my knowledge and provides a valuable resource to women everywhere. Thanks to them for joining me in helping the planet be a softer, more accepting and loving place to be.

All of my friends, colleagues, and clients who continue to support me in my quest for helping women achieve authentic sexual connection.

To my two nieces, Julia and Kayla, who inspire me to carry on so that they may grow up in a safer, more accepting, sensual world.

And finally, buckets full of thanks to my dear, sweet husband, Barry, for believing in me, picking up all of the slack while I work, and mostly, for showing me that love is ever evolving, ever growing, and always a worthwhile adventure.

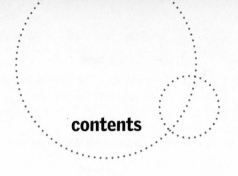

contents

introduction

Tough times shouldn't slow down your sex life. Whether you're stressed at work, worried about global warming, concerned about the stock market, anxious about your bills, or frustrated with your kids, great sex with your partner shouldn't fall off your priority list.

The truth is, stress will likely be present in all of our lives in one form or another; global warming and frustration with work or the government will likely stick around over the course of our lifetimes. The important thing is not to let these things get in the way of living and enjoying life. Equally important is that you find simple ways to improve your quality of life, because negative news and situations can and will impact your outlook and your mental and physical health. That's where this book steps in: this book will help you manage and banish the stress of hard times in the most fun way possible—with great sex!

A great sex life makes absolutely everything else easier to deal with, whether it's handling money issues or multitasking at work. Being satisfied with the passion and love you have in your life allows you the space and ability to focus on and improve other areas. Meanwhile, getting a regular dose of endorphins will have you on a natural high and feeling good about your partner. And when your friends, your family, and especially your children see you connected, loving toward your partner, and happy, a domino effect is created: those around you start to feel happy and less stressed.

Studies have proven that regular, first-rate sex will help you live longer. Sex also acts as a pain reliever and as an antihistamine to unblock a stuffy nose, and can help you sleep, burn calories, and clean your pores, making your skin glow. What more do you need to feel terrific? Visualize how wonderful your life will be when you are walking around with a twinkle in your eye and a glow in your cheeks and you are truly happy.

But perhaps you don't need me to convince you that you should be having great sex. Perhaps you already desire to boost the bounce in your bedroom and are turning to this book for great ideas from a professional who is skilled in the area of sex. If you want to discover who you are as a sexual woman, I can lend a hand. My skill as a sex coach is helping women discover their inner sensuality. I help women bring it out into their lives in the way that works best for them. Helping you discover your authentic sensual self is what I consider my gift.

As you read through this guide, you'll share in the experiences of six women who, like you, wish to create a little more excitement in their bedrooms. If you're like Michelle, whose desire isn't what it used to be now that she's perimenopausal and a little overweight, the titillating ideas in this book will get those romantic juices flowing again. Yoko wants to keep her current spark alive, but with the business she and her new husband are starting, it's a challenge. Maybe, like Alison, you've almost given up getting to the next level of lovemaking in your relationship. Juanita oozes confidence at work and out in the world, but when she walks through the bedroom door, she turns into an insecure schoolgirl. She's frustrated because she hasn't yet had her first orgasm. See how she blossoms with simple baby steps.

I've read a lot of sex books that have some fantastic suggestions for ways to rev your engine, but the ideas usually involve steps that simply aren't doable for most of us. Consider the unreasonable scenarios for those who can't afford to run off for the weekend or charge expensive items like lingerie, rose petals, fancy scents, and caviar to their credit cards, as well as the multitude of sex positions that aren't realistic for the average woman or man, positions requiring flexibility and assertiveness that a lot of us haven't yet mastered. A rewarding sex life shouldn't break the bank or the back!

After reading this book you will know how to bring your erotic nature a little closer to the surface; you will have the tools in your hand to maintain intimacy, turn on your inner sensual side, and create the love life you've always dreamed of. I wrote this book for the discerning woman who respects herself and her partner and wants more in life and from love. A woman who appreciates that value and cost do not go hand in hand. A woman who understands that life's stressful moments necessitate intimacy, passion, and great sex.

Great Sex for Hard Times will show you that it's easy to set up wonderfully simple, fun, and amazingly intimate and sexy moments that will carry you through the hard times and bring about your very best times!

Passionately,
Kim Switnicki, ECPC, ACC
Sex educator, speaker, and sex and intimacy coach

chapter 1

Welcome to Sexual Satisfaction

And the day came when the risk to remain tight in a bud was more painful than the risk it took to blossom. —Anaïs Nin, author

Hot, steamy, sweaty passion. Do you remember the last time you had great sex? Remember how the passion flowed and you let yourself go, completely taking in every scent, every breath, and every beat of your heart? Did you ooze sexuality, sensuality, and animal lust? Were you wild with abandon and inhibition free? Perhaps this passionate event was in your bedroom, or maybe it was in another room of the house—a kitchen perhaps, or on the stairs, because you didn't quite make it up to the bedroom. Possibly the moment was so intense you kept the lights on and didn't even care what angle your lover saw you from because everything felt so deliciously fantastic that you couldn't bear the thought of stopping for even a few seconds.

"Yes, take me, I'm yours!" is all you thought and felt. You heard sexy moans and even growls coming from between your lips. The scream building inside you bubbled up from your very core and you *knew* you'd see fireworks this time. When the pivotal moment came for you to fully let go and dive over the cliff into your exquisite climax, you tackled it with a running leap and soared over the edge.

The bliss afterward was heavenly and you sensually licked your lips and asked him, "When will you be ready for round two, my love?"

If you've never had mind-numbing sex that sent you to paradise, don't worry. It may not happen overnight, but don't despair—the idea of it happening for you isn't a pipe dream! You've taken one step by picking up this book. And over the next twenty chapters you will receive fun tips, tricks, and techniques that can get you there one step at a time! But before we explore how to activate all your hot zones and seduce your lover, let me briefly explain why great sex should be a priority in your life and how to best use this book.

> ♥ If you put as much time, energy, attention, and commitment into your sex life as you do into your job or other areas of your life—you'll notice a huge difference in your whole life.

Great Sex Boosts Your Confidence

If you remember the last time you had great sex and how incredible you felt, think about how nice it would be to have that feeling more often. Recall how people around you have responded to you after you've had a particularly spectacular evening. What sort of mood are you in after great lovemaking? Yoko says,

The girls in the office seem to always know when Jim and I have had a hot night, because the next day all I get are smiles, knowing looks, and a chorus of "How are YOU doing this morning, Yoko?" It's safe to say that there must be a twinkle in my eye and a bounce in my step that people can see!

Practice making love more and you will boost your confidence in ways you haven't even thought of yet. The more comfortable you are making love and exploring and receiving pleasure, the more likely you are to get creative, be adventurous, and start having loads of fun in and out of the bedroom. You may even start doing it with the lights on or become totally comfortable in any position, no matter how exposed you are. The more fun sex you have, the better you feel about yourself. The better you feel about yourself, the more sure you are and the more likely you are to initiate sex and even enjoy it more. If you're enjoying it more, you'll probably do it more. Can you see the positive, upward spiral of how more great sex equals even more great sex? Can you see how the more great sex you have, the more confident you will become? And this doesn't apply to just feeling confident in the context of making love; you'll start to feel more confident in general.

Great Sex Makes You Feel More Sensual and Sexy

Once you decide you want more fabulous sex in your life, set an intention. Be deliberate about it and decide to pay some real attention to your love life. People often speak of setting goals for their finances or in business or even for other dreams, yet they rarely set intentions for their love life. Once you decide a great sex life is important and necessary to your satisfaction with your life *and* you decide to do something about it, change will happen. Some changes will be subtle, such as noticing sexy things about your mate that you may have ignored before but that now pop out at you. Some may be remarkable, such as feeling turned on a whole lot more and being suddenly willing to try new things that you were nervous about in the past. Telling your mind that you want more sex will allow you the ability to seize opportunities or create occasions for great sex right in your bedroom. Just like when you buy a red car and then suddenly notice other red cars everywhere, your mind will recognize the limitless sexy opportunities much more often.

Once you start seeing opportunities and acting on them (since you have created them for yourself!), you will notice an amazing thing. Because you have this sexy new mind-set, you will find yourself becoming more sensual with everything you do. *You will feel sexier.* Your sex appeal will be quite naturally boosted because of this new erotic energy you are emitting, and people around you will notice. You may:

- walk taller, which helps you look slimmer and more shapely.
- stand more sensually while waiting in line, instead of slumping.
- engage in more direct eye contact with people you encounter in your day, especially the cute ones!
- do naturally flirty things such as tossing your hair, licking your lips, or casually caressing your neck while chatting with a cute server or flight attendant.

When you invite your sexuality into your life fully, you will be rewarded with wolf calls, flirty comments, and a stimulated sex drive. You can be sure that a "headache" will never again stand in the way of your having sex. Can you handle more of that in your day? I sure hope so.

Great Sex Is Vital to Healthy Living

Stress can age us and wreak havoc on our immune systems, but great sex can reduce stress and its negative effects on the body. Dr. Mehmet Oz of Oprah Winfrey fame has quoted a Duke University study saying that engaging in regular, loving, monogamous sex will help keep your body younger and more healthy. If you increase the amount of sex you have, you will live longer. Studies continue to prove this over and over!

Regular sex has been known to lower blood pressure, improve cardiovascular health, burn calories, and increase the amount of Immunoglobulin A, an antibody that fights off colds. Kissing alone is excellent for oral hygiene, as the saliva generated from kissing helps remove plaque from your teeth and promotes healthy gums. The bonus is that if you improve your overall health you will naturally boost your libido or sex drive. How lucky for us that sex makes us healthier and that being healthier makes us hornier. It stands to reason then: better sex equals a better life.

Great Sex Elevates Your Mood and Improves Your Mind

Oxytocin and endorphins are released into your system when you have sex and act as a relaxer and a pain reliever, respectively. When you are relaxed and calm, you can be more present for conversations and for moments with family and friends, which will create a domino effect. When you're a joy to be around and everyone loves to be in your presence, their days will be impacted as well. They too benefit when they come away from an interaction with you and they feel great. Then their good moods help the people they encounter in their days. . . . Your having great sex helps everyone you meet have better days and they help others have good days and so on and so on.

Sex also creates more blood flow to the brain, which is linked to improved memory. Dr. Daniel G. Amen, author of *Change Your Brain, Change Your Life*, says, "Enhancing estrogen levels for women through regular sexual activity enhances overall brain activity and improves memory." Now, there's something you might have taken for granted: a healthy sex life makes for a healthy brain.

Great Sex Improves Your Emotional Connection

Authentic connection between two loving adults is never stronger than when they make love, except perhaps during the birth of a child—and how did that come about anyhow? The embrace of a lover makes us feel good. It reassures us that we are desirable, wanted, and cared for. One of our purposes on the planet is to love and to be loved and there is no stronger way to show that love than to make love. You often hear stories of people who, when faced with an immediate, life-threatening situation, will have a hankering for some loving. It seems that sexual play is a life-affirming activity, but let's not wait until we're faced with certain death to enjoy it! It's also worth noting that oxytocin, which acts as a relaxer, also promotes feelings of love and bonding, which bring you and your partner together.

Great Sex Promotes a Healthy Relationship

Lovemaking should be an accepted part of a healthy, loving relationship between adults. Displays of romance in your relationship are a great opportunity for kids to see sexuality positively, which provides a solid basis for them to become well-adjusted adults. No need to invite them into your bedroom, but don't hide the fact that Mom and Dad have quiet time for themselves alone and it is cherished by both of you.

Have Great Sex All the Time

We now may be with the same person for forty, fifty, or sixty years. As recently as a hundred years ago we didn't even live that long! Good sex is vital to a relationship, and variety can be critical to good sex. These pages will guide you to up the variety scale to keep your love flame burning brightly and your relationship from entering Dullsville. If you're in a new relationship and want to keep it from getting stale, then start from a position of strength and build from there.

Sex is not the absolute and only thing that will keep your relationships strong. Compatibility and communication are what last and carry you through the long term. However, great sex can carry you through the rough spots and can help to keep the bond of intimacy strong so you don't end up feeling as though you are in a relationship with a sibling. Now is your chance to lose the stress in your life and turn all that anxious energy into something wild and passionate in your bedroom. We will cover various aspects of a solid, healthy sexual relationship and give you the means to develop your relationship so you're hot for your best friend. How powerful and exciting is that?

Deeper satisfaction comes from pushing and exploring your

sexual boundaries. Do this while also respecting your partner's boundaries and you will be rewarded with a lifetime of hotter sex. Expand your horizons just a little with new positions (see chapters 9 and 10), variety in your locations (see chapters 4, 15, and 17), and even the times of day you choose to have your fun. Won't your sweetheart be thrilled when you start doing things you have previously only done in your fantasies? Combine these simple ideas with better communication and you have a recipe for sizzling sex that will continue to surprise you both for the rest of your lives.

Situations change. If you tried something in the past and it didn't work out as well as you'd hoped it would and it still intrigues you, give it another chance. You may have been with a different partner or your hormones may have been at a different level or the environment just may not have been right at the time. Our bodies change so much as we age that what was uncomfortable once may now be lovely! You may discover that you now love doggy-style sex or that anal play is really quite fun. You may rediscover your G-spot after years of thinking it had disappeared. With your current partner, a blindfold may add just the right touch of mystery to release all of your inhibitions. Revelations will occur for you throughout your sexual life as long as you step out of that stale place and keep exploring. This book is the perfect tool for taking action immediately to create spectacular sexual activity in your life.

How to Use This Guide

Creative, daring and, adventurous. These are the qualities I suspect you have if you've read this far. You may feel you've forgotten that you have them, but they're still there! For ease of writing I'm also assuming you are a heterosexual woman and you have a man in your life. This way I can keep the pronouns simple. But please note: if you are not heterosexual or you are a straight man, you will still discover some wild and remarkable secrets, some great tips for romance, and some new ways to please the special person in your life!

How do you use this book? There is no wrong way to enjoy it. You can certainly read it from cover to cover to give you a solid picture of what you want to create for yourself, but that isn't required or even recommended. The chapters are set up so you can pick one, read through it, and add some spice immediately. Or you can flip through and select a few Quickie Tips, such as the following one, which offers simple and easy ideas on how to create a more sensual environment or a more sensual you.

●●● Kim's **QUICKIE TIP**

Recall or write out all the reasons you got together with your sweetie. Revisit that space you once held for putting him above all others. When you need inspiration for your day or you simply want to feel wonderful and escape from whatever is ailing or worrying you, go back in time and remember some of the fun things you did when you first started dating. It's much better for you than a drink, and likely more fun too!

You'll also encounter some tips on how to add some excitement to the bedroom at little or no cost to you. My Cash-Saver Tips are ways you can add sizzle with minimal resources.

$ $ $ Kim's **CASH-SAVER TIP**

Pick up fancy notepaper from a dollar store to write out sexy, memorable invitations. Get creative with craft or scrapbooking bits you may have lying about the house, and start thinking, "How can I make this into a sexy coupon or an invitation for adult playtime?"

The Sexy Challenges I've included throughout the book are fun and will ensure your success in upping the sizzle factor in your sex life. They are in-depth ways to get the most from what you learn in each chapter. Undertaking them also shows a commitment to your sexual relationship. I've set up the Sexy Challenges so you can see at a glance the items required, the preparation time, and the special features of the challenge, such as:

- ❍ the cost range
- ❍ the challenge raciness factor (either Regular, Bold, or Extreme)
- ❍ the main benefit, such as: Improves Communication, Reduces Inhibitions, Develops Intimacy, Improves Sexual Skills, or Increases Inner Sensuality

Look at these challenges as an assortment of stimulating dares to help you experiment with new skills, talents, and techniques so you can become the lover of your dreams. Your first challenge awaits you at the end of this chapter.

We each have our own pace when it comes to sexual exploration. Baby steps are usually safest and will most likely keep you moving forward. For some, like Marcia, you may want to find new ways to set off the fireworks sooner rather than later, so you might pick a chapter or two that calls out to you and set something up for tonight, tomorrow, and possibly the next night. Perhaps, like Marcia, you want to start having fun again because you feel the pressure of time; to help make ends meet, Marcia will soon be going back to work after staying at home for the past ten years raising her three lovely kids, and she wants to take advantage of the time she has now.

Pick up the book whenever you feel the urge to add a slice

of fun to your day or evening! In fact, in responding to that urge, you'll likely be introducing some spontaneity, which can be the single greatest trick for having a marvelously fun sex life. Planting the 10-Second Kiss when he least expects it (chapter 6), wrapping him in a snuggly towel when he steps out of the shower (chapter 15), or offering him a sexy coupon (chapter 20) that he can use immediately may be all you need to send your love life from a ho-hum three out of ten to a scorching twelve out of ten on the heat scale.

Men love spontaneity. You can simply leave the book on the nightstand or in the bathroom for your lover to read with a Post-it or two marking things you wish to try right away.

💜 Sex is a fabulous pastime that is invigorating and feels incredible. So grab your zest for life, put sex on the front burner, and let's get cooking!

SEXY CHALLENGE
Three Times for Luck

You'll Need: Paper, a pen, Post-its
Prep Time: 5 to 15 minutes (depending on your creative spark)
Cost: $0–$5
Raciness Factor: Regular
Benefit: Improves Communication

Come up with three ways to pass along your newfound sexual curiosity (for example, this book!) to your lover in a romantic way. Here is a sample note you can leave for him. You may even seal it with a lipstick imprint or spray a bit of his favorite perfume on the note. Use the following to stir up your own imagination:

Tonight is the beginning of a sensual adventure you won't soon forget. I want to give you something sexy, new, and exciting so you realize how much you mean to me. Get ready for some steam in the bedroom, darling!

Perhaps you can mark certain pages with Post-it notes or a highlighter; photocopy pages and leave them under his pillow or in his briefcase; send him an e-mail with excerpts from the book and leave the book in a conspicuous place, like the bathroom counter while he's in the shower, so he sees it before coming to bed; or try writing your own addition to a chapter and insert the pages, asking him to check it over for "typos" while you get ready for bed.

The most important thing to remember with all of the information, suggestions, and ideas you'll find in this book is to have a fabulous time! Laugh, smile, enjoy, and push yourself a tiny bit each time you try something, and you'll find success. Use this as an opportunity to sex up your life and expand your sensuality and you'll enjoy the many physical and emotional rewards—and so will your man!

chapter 2

How Your Mind and Body Figure into the Mix

An orgasm a day keeps the doctor away. —Mae West, actress

Not all men are from Mars and not all women are from Venus. Misunderstanding occurs when you try to slot people into boxes that restrict their behavior, and suppose or assume that they should behave in a certain way. If you read or hear about how "all" men behave and how "all" women feel—and believe it— you run the risk of adding unnecessary confusion to your relationship. Some people theorize that men express their emotions by engaging in sex and that women need to feel emotionally connected in order to have sex. This simply isn't true for everyone, and one cannot afford to accept generalizations as truths!

As humans we operate within such an incredible range of emotions and behaviors. Our behaviors alter as we mature and as we enter into different relationships. In a healthy relationship there is a natural flow of energy and power, and it isn't simply that the woman has all the feminine energy and the man has all the masculine energy. We all possess both energies, yet one is more prominent in each of us. I carry a lot of masculine energy and am usually direct and assertive. My husband has a fabulous feminine energy and his sensitivity is part of what drew me to him. He is also very male—comfortable with a chainsaw in his hands, rock climbing, or rescuing people in stormy seas with the Coast Guard Auxiliary. If we've been fighting, we don't have make-up sex to connect because my husband needs to feel that we are emotionally connecting before we engage physically. On the other hand, I don't necessarily have to feel loving to have a romp in the sheets.

Be aware of your own unique needs and don't ever assume that your partner is a "typical" male. He is unique, and learning how to communicate with him and finding out exactly what is on his mind will serve you better than any book to guide you on his actions.

Introduction to Sex

When we're young we become "hardwired" for a lot of the things that will please us sexually. Perhaps when you were a child you had your first masturbatory experience while you were hiding in a closet and there happened to be a leather coat hanging up above you and you could smell it and feel it resting on your shoulder as you had this lovely, sensual experience of your first self-pleasured orgasm. It is logical to think that you will be turned on by the thought of leather against your skin. The trick is not to fight it, but to use it to your advantage. It's not likely that you can *only* receive pleasure if leather is involved (that's more like a fetish) but rather that you really get turned on when leather is near you. Get yourself a gorgeous leather corset or a leather pillow for your bed, or buy your man a leather jacket.

When Marcia learned about hardwired turn-ons, she was so relieved!

> When I was younger, I had a babysitter who used to have boyfriends over when she babysat us. One night I snuck out of bed because I heard some strange sounds coming from downstairs. There was this lace curtain my mother was repairing draped from a hook on the wall at the top of the stairs. I hid behind the curtain and peered through the tiny holes down into the living room at my babysitter and her boyfriend having sex on our couch. I had a bird's-eye view! I didn't really know what was happening, but I saw him on top of her and knew it was wrong what they were doing. I was also very aroused and mesmerized watching them.
>
> I used to think I was some sort of pervert because I get so turned on whenever I see lace. Now I have two beautiful lace-covered pillows on my bed so they are near me when we make love. Don doesn't know the story behind the pillows, and for now I'm happy with my harmless secret weapon to rev me up whenever I need some help.

Being Present

Emotions live in the brain (and new research suggests they are also in the stomach) and the brain is the most important sexual organ that we women have. The skin is probably the *largest* sexual organ, and we'll talk later about the pleasures of touch. Have you ever had an orgasm in your dreams? We all have the ability to have an orgasm without any physical stimulation at all. I know a woman who taught herself to orgasm through med-itation. It took her three years, but she can do it with ease now. That's dedication! Your mind is incredibly powerful—when you tap into that power, you can have wildly passionate sexual expe-riences every time. We have the power to orgasm just thinking sexual thoughts. I love that possibility.

One of the complexities of female sexuality is that the amygdala in a woman's brain needs to be shut off in order for her to become aroused and reach the peak of orgasm. The amygdala is engaged when you are stressed and worried about something. If you are thinking of what you need to remember to ask the doctor next week or how you're going to pay for your child's education, it isn't possible to get turned on, let alone climax. There really isn't any mystery here.

One secret to help shut down the amygdala is to keep your-self warm. A hot bath before lovemaking, a warm bedroom, and nice, comfy, warm blankets are great ideas to help you get your body temperature up to hot-sex level.

Another trick is to have your feet rubbed. This also has been shown to turn off the amygdala and get women ready to be turned on. Juanita doesn't like her feet touched because she's ticklish, so she started asking her man to massage her hands. She can now more easily let the strain of her day drift away with a five-minute hand massage. Plus it gets her into love mode much faster.

●●● Kim's **QUICKIE TIP**

Play footsies with your man at dinner to signal that you'd like a foot rub. Once he realizes that this often puts you in the mood for more than washing dishes, you'll find him eager.

Four-Stage Cycle

Your sexual response occurs in a four-stage cycle as you go through arousal and the release of orgasm. We experience:

- Excitement
- Plateau
- Orgasm
- Resolution

There are slight differences between men and women during these stages. Both experience the heart pumping faster, increasing blood flow, which engorges all the important parts like lips, nipples, and genitals, and causes our skin to flush with a rosy hue. Just think, if we stayed aroused all the time, we wouldn't need makeup! We also experience muscle tension, and our bodies become toasty warm. Women also start to get wet vaginally (lubrication) and the vagina swells and tips back, shifting the uterus and the cervix to accommodate full penetration. In men, the testicles rise up toward the body and the scrotum will contract.

The Plateau stage is essentially a heightening of excitement. The female clitoris may retract under the clitoral hood (see the diagram in the next chapter) and men may emit "precome," fluid from the tip of the penis (see the diagram in the next chapter).

Technically orgasm is the release and letting go of built-up erotic tension. This occurs through involuntary muscle contractions—you can't stop it once it begins! There are between three and fifteen contractions, so having toned pelvic-floor muscles enhances orgasm strength for men and women.

Men experience a point of no return right before orgasm but women *do not*. Ladies need that perfect stimulation speed, angle, and pressure right up to and even during our orgasmic contractions. This is a fundamental difference that bears conversation to ensure that you are both aware of each other's needs. As for your man, you also want to learn whether he likes stimulation to continue, slow down, speed up, or stop completely during his orgasm.

●●● Kim's **QUICKIE TIP**

To learn what he likely prefers when you are stimulating him to orgasm with your mouth or hands, pay attention to what he does during his climax when you have intercourse. Does he stay still or continue moving? This isn't an absolute answer, and it also may vary for him, but it's a good start.

During the final phase of resolution, everything returns to the normal state before arousal. If you didn't achieve orgasmic release, this stage may take a bit longer. If Yoko makes love and doesn't orgasm (which is rare), she shares this technique:

I love to shower after we make love, and when I wash myself between my legs, I enjoy feeling the swelling and juiciness of it. Sometimes it turns me on and I end up playing with myself in the shower. For those times, I usually call Jim in to join me, and he will hold me while I do it. It's very romantic!

Desire is considered by some experts to be an additional phase, and it may occur at any point in the cycle. I would also add Anticipation, which can more easily lead to Desire. Be on the lookout throughout the book for the many opportunities to build anticipation into your romantic life. The beautiful thing about sexuality is the complexity, mystery, and delicious fluidity of it all.

Foreplay Secrets

Foreplay is crucial for women's bodies to be prepared for great sex. When you add in the element of anticipation, which is something done entirely by you, your partner has less "work" to do. This is especially helpful for quickie sex (see chapter 16). However, if you make time for funky foreplay and really get into the sheer joy of exploring each others' bodies, it can turn ordinary sex into extraordinary sex. Remember that foreplay is not just the play that happens in bed before you have intercourse. It begins at the beginning of your day when you take time for a ten-second snuggle-up and a whispered "I love you," or "Hope your day is fabulous," or the more enticing "Can't wait till we meet back here again tonight!" Look for as many openings as you can (in the shower, at breakfast, during coffee break phone calls, in e-mails, at impromptu lunches) to let your partner know you desire him and find him sexy. It will make you feel warm and delicious as well. Throughout this book are ways to help you keep those foreplay fires burning all through the day. This way, when the time comes to engage in hot sex—you are ready because you've been priming the pump all day.

Foreplay is an art, and if you treat it as a lusty experiment to see how long you can tease each other before you practically beg for satisfaction, you will both win. Look upon your partner as though you have just seen his luscious body naked for the first time. Explore every nook, cranny, and crevice with new eyes, lips, tongue, fingers, etc. Having your bodies prepared for intercourse will make that experience much more enjoyable for you both. Then watch out for fireworks!

Why Foreplay?

Pleasure for you both should be the main focus when you make love. One way to ensure pleasure during intercourse is to be sure you are fully prepared. By this I mean that you are aroused so that your vagina has swelled and shifted and that you are moist and slippery. If you have penetration—whether by finger, toy, or penis—and you aren't lubricated, you may feel some discomfort. This can set up a negative mind–body connection that can lead to problems in the future. If you try to attempt penetration into a dry vagina, you can cause tiny tears that you may not see or feel. They won't necessarily bleed, but they can create a breeding ground for bacteria, so stay slippery! There are many reasons for women to be dry even though they are aroused. You may be drier than usual due to:

- hormonal changes (due to surgery, menstruation, giving birth, breast-feeding, menopause, medications)
- stress
- fatigue
- alcohol consumption
- aging (vaginal walls become thinner and secretions diminish)
- drugs (over the counter or illicit)

Even something as common as allergy medication can cause trouble since it dries up mucous membranes and you have mucous membranes between your legs! Check with your healthcare provider if you're concerned about any medications, so you don't think there's a problem with your libido when there isn't.

Lubricant

Lubricant is the single most important sexual accessory to have in your collection. Having super-slipperiness during penetration offers many benefits:

- More pleasure for you, with slippery surfaces rubbing against each other
- More pleasure for your partner (see above)
- Minimal risk of tearing
- Longer periods of intercourse than usual before irritation
- The clitoris may need lubrication, and natural lubrication may not spread to the clitoris (some women prefer slippery contact over friction on their clitoris—feel free to experiment with both options)
- The body is encouraged to open up, creating a more positive experience than if you are dry and attempting penetration
- The G-spot area can be more easily detected by a slippery finger (see chapter 10)

You can't be too juicy! If you aren't a big fan, though, and you like more friction, then having a cloth handy is a simple solution. I'm a huge fan of flavored lubricant, and I'll discuss types of lubricants in chapter 15.

SEXY CHALLENGE
Funky Footsies

You'll Need: Lotion, a warm room
Prep Time: 1 minute (to put out the invitation—remember to make it sexy)

Cost: $0
Raciness Factor: Regular
Benefit: Increases Inner Sensuality

Invite your lover to trade foot rubs with you. Pick a time when you have at least an hour free and rub his feet first for at least fifteen minutes. You can wash them in the tub first or take a shower together (bonus points for this) so you are both squeaky clean. Make sure the heat is up in the room so you are warm. When it's your turn, lie back if possible and fantasize about what images, sights, smells, tastes, materials, or whatever it is that really turns you on. Let your mind wander as your feet are massaged and notice how quickly you can relax into a more sensual state when you are present and enjoying the sensation of his hands caressing your feet. If you discover something in your fantasy that really turns you on, think about how you will incorporate it into your lovemaking.

chapter **3**

Your Delicious Body, Created for
Amazing Sexual Pleasure

When the authorities warn you of the dangers of having sex,
there is an important lesson to be learned. Do not have sex
with the authorities. —**Matt Groening, creator of** *The Simpsons*

Viva la vulva! Likely the most misunderstood, mis-
named, and maligned part of our anatomy, the vulva
is essentially all of the outer female genitalia and is
often mistakenly called the vagina. The vagina is the
tube-shaped passageway to the reproductive organs
and is inside the body, while the vulva represents the
outside of our female core. Rejoice in this lovely
treasure since yours is unique in this world. Our vul-
vas can be different colors, shapes, and sizes, and can
have different levels of sensitivity.

At the top we have the mound of Venus (mons
pubis or mons veneris), which has pubic hair and is
really a fleshy pad protecting the pubic bone. The
outer lips (labia majora) typically have hair on them,
are fleshy, and can be mottled in color or even a dif-

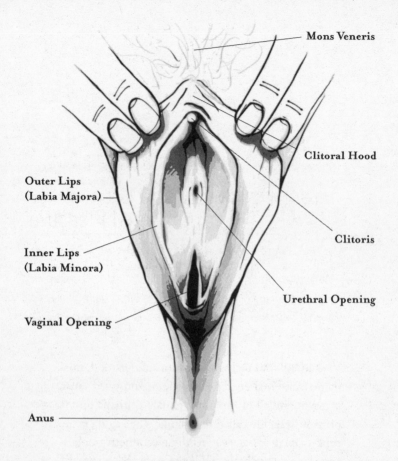

Mons Veneris

Clitoral Hood

Outer Lips
(Labia Majora)

Inner Lips
(Labia Minora)

Clitoris

Vaginal Opening

Urethral Opening

Anus

ferent color from the inner lips (labia minora). The inner lips are hairless, usually thinner, and sometimes seem larger or longer than the outer lips. Where they join at the top is the magical head (glans) of the clitoris. This is what I call the tip of the clitoral iceberg. Due to its sensitivity, it requires a protective hood. We'll cover the clitoris in more detail soon. Below the clitoris is the urethral opening, where we urinate from and where we can ejaculate from (see chapter 10 to read all about ejaculation).

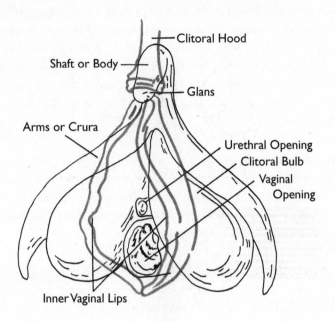

Shaft or Body — Clitoral Hood

Glans

Arms or Crura

Urethral Opening
Clitoral Bulb
Vaginal Opening

Inner Vaginal Lips

Below this is the opening to the vagina. The area between here and the anus is the perineum, which is loaded with nerves and often gets overlooked during sexual play.

●●● Kim's **QUICKIE TIP**

Try to incorporate the fun zone (perineum) in your next lovemaking session by encouraging your honey to use his fingers or tongue to rub, squeeze, or lick it for some titillating pleasure.

Unique to women, the clitoris is the only part of the human anatomy designed strictly for sexual pleasure. It is the source of much mystery for both men and women, and most believe it is only the tiny nub that we feel at the top of the vulva. In fact, it is a large and complex organ with a series of nerves spreading deep into the vagina, nerves that only recently have been mapped out! The body of the clitoris goes down behind the pubic bone by about three inches, and the clitoral bulbs are analogous to the testicles on a man. The arms (crura) curve down on either side of the vaginal opening, which accounts for the pleasure Alison feels:

> *Whenever Bill plays with my clitoris or puts his fingers inside me, he sometimes flicks my pussy lips and it sends jolts of pleasure right through me. I'm not sure if he does it on purpose because he can tell I love it or it's just a fluke, but I love it when it happens.*

A lot of women enjoy having their vaginal lips played with because they are like a tuning fork, sending pleasure waves right up to the head of the clitoris, which has *eight thousand nerve endings!* This is the most concentrated number of nerves in all of human anatomy. Since the clitoris is so sensitive, it has a protective hood or fold of skin covering it. If this hood weren't there, we likely couldn't wear snug pants or else we'd spend all of our time having orgasms and never get anything done. Some of us have a tiny hood and others have many layers or folds covering the glans. When aroused, the clitoris is usually much easier to find, since it actually gets an erection and peeks out from under the hood. As we get closer to our peaks, it often retreats. This makes it challenging for your lover to manually stimulate you when his target keeps moving! This is why communication with your lover is vital for you to receive exactly what you need for orgasm.

There are an infinite number of ways to please a clitoris. You can apply hard or soft pressure, use dry friction or have slippery slickness, go around in circles or rub up and down or any of the variations in between. You may discover your secret to erotic bliss is light pressure from the tip of a tongue, or perhaps you prefer the strong pulses of a vibrator or strong fingers rubbing back and forth. Some women don't even like direct attention on the clitoris, preferring indirect stimulation instead, achieved by squeezing the clitoris between the vaginal lips or even rubbing along the side or near the base of the clitoris and not right on the tip. Find out what rocks your world and pass along your magic tricks to your honey so he can be a magician in the bedroom.

The core to a man's sexual identity is of course the magnificent penis shown on page 28. This image is of a circumcised man and is also how an uncircumcised man will look when erect. The tiny opening at the tip (meatus) is where the pre-come fluid, the ejaculate, and urine all exit. This small hole is tender, so lick it with care and never try to insert even your tongue inside it unless you are super-gentle or your man asks you to. Next we have the head of the penis (glans), which is similar to the head of the clitoris and is extremely sensitive. The corona is the ridge that encircles the head and is a great guide during oral sex for indicating that your mouth is just about at the end of the penis if your eyes are closed! Just beneath this ridge at the front is the magic spot called the frenulum. This band of tissue is super-receptive to concentrated tongue action during oral sex. Do this and you'll have a friend for life. Some men can even orgasm having a vibrator held here!

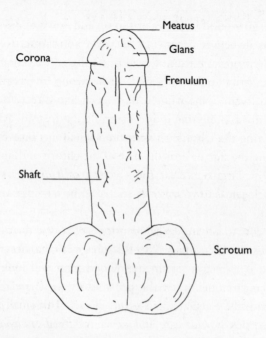

The shaft is often curved slightly and brings lots of pleasure when stroked. Not all men can orgasm with only shaft play, so be sure to include the head for the full-pleasure effect. Next we have the scrotum, which holds two testicles. This sac is super-responsive, so tread lightly. Gentle licking, caressing, and slight tugging can make him putty in your hands, and I'm not talking about his erection, since it's bound to just get harder! Below the scrotum is the perineum, which runs all the way to the anus, just as in women. Loaded with nerve endings, this area is erotically charged, so experiment and drive him wild.

$ $ $ Kim's **CASH-SAVER TIP**

Ordinary dish soap or hand soap can be used for bath bubbles, so you can indulge in a tub for two where washing each others' backs can take all night. . . . Light a few candles for some added romance.

Jen recalls the day she chose to worship Lionel's penis:

We've been together since college and know each other so well that it's hard to find anything new to do in bed. The last time we made love I decided to completely focus on Lionel and his penis. I went down on him right away and really took my time. I was thinking of it as a scrumptious delight that I just couldn't get enough of. It turned me on so much watching him moan, and he was so blissed out. I couldn't believe how wet I got watching him. Every now and then he would open his eyes, and that made me a bit self-conscious, but mostly he laid back and he seemed to enjoy it so much.

I stopped before he came and got up and straddled him. He seemed a bit shocked at that, and also because I was so wet. It didn't take more than five or six strokes before I could feel my own orgasm coming. It was pretty powerful thinking about how much I loved him and how hot things still could be. Wow. What a night.

Be willing to try new things and be open to a variety of ways to please your man, whether with different strokes, mouth moves, lovemaking positions, temperature sensations, or simply doing things you don't normally do. Mainly you want to be gentle with the penis and learn what pressure and grip he likes and go from there. My favorite way to do this is to watch him please himself. This only covers the manual portion of the show, but it's a great start!

Male Sexual Challenges

If your man has any concerns with premature ejaculation or erectile function, see your healthcare provider since there are medical conditions and medications that may be a contributing factor. Once these have been ruled out, there are some alternatives to drugs that should be explored first.

Fun techniques such as the squeeze technique work well for premature ejaculation. Essentially you and your man employ the technique of squeezing the penis with a thumb and two fingers at the base or at the frenulum when he is close to but has not yet reached the point of no return, to prevent him from climaxing. He can do this on his own when he masturbates as well to prolong that experience. What great homework! There is also a desensitizing gel (available from my Web site at www.kimswitnicki.com/greatsexforhardtimes) that you can use as a temporary fix to break the cycle of quick orgasm. It numbs him slightly where applied so he can last longer. I recommend the gel as a first step but urge you to work toward a full experience of all sexual sensations.

For erectile difficulties you can use a simple erection ring (also available at my website), which is applied once the penis is erect. It helps keep the erection by restricting blood flow back into the body. Penis pumps can also help if there is difficulty achieving an erection. They work using suction to bring blood flow to the area. There are many good choices online, or you can e-mail me directly for more information at kim@kimswitnicki.com.

Patience is the key with any difficulty either of you is having. Communication is also crucial so that you continue to support each other toward a healthy, loving sexual relationship.

Note: Throughout the book I will refer to resources and products to assist you on your journey. A special Web page has been created listing all of the references in the book to make it easier for you to find what you want. Lioness for Lovers is a division of my company that provides adult toys hand-selected by me and also produces some of my books, audios, and other products I have created. I look forward to serving you in whatever way I can.

Orgasm

Multiple orgasms simply refers to more than one orgasm in a lovemaking session. They aren't necessarily one right after another. It is a rare woman who can handle any stimulation of her clitoris immediately following an orgasm. Most of us need a brief rest due to hypersensitivity, and then we can build up sensation and reach our peak again and can do this repeatedly. We can actually build to stronger and stronger orgasms each time in a session. Men, on the other hand, tend to get less intense orgasms as the session progresses.

After he ejaculates, there is a "refractory" period where he needs time to be able to have another erection. This period can be fifteen minutes for teens and up to several hours for older men. Both sexes tend to experience hypersensitivity right after an orgasm and don't watch any touching! Some men don't even want the penis touched during their orgasms, while most women like you to keep doing exactly what you were doing during their orgasm.

💜 Orgasm shouldn't be the goal or focus of lovemaking—even with self-pleasure. Discovering what pleases you, enjoying being in the moment while engaged in sexual play, and connecting in an intimate, honest way with your lover is the real challenge. Go for it!

Michelle has been married for twenty-two years. Between being anxious about her financial future, being perimenopausal, and helping her daughter navigate her first pregnancy, she is tired and has lost interest in sex:

> *I haven't had an orgasm in quite a few years. My vaginal dryness, weight gain, and the fact that my husband, Dave, just doesn't look at me that way anymore all mean sex is the last thing on my mind.*
>
> *I tried this challenge and was surprised because it seemed like forever since I'd had anything sensual in my life. I don't even know the last time I looked at myself like that. I felt empowered and more in control. I don't know if I have any of that erotic energy yet, but I'm going to get some lubricant and might start masturbating again. Let's give this a shot!*

SEXY CHALLENGE
Sensual Solitary Celebration

You'll Need: Bubble bath, body lotion, mirror, drink, paper, and pen
Prep Time: None
Cost: $0–$5
Raciness Factor: Bold
Benefit: Increases Inner Sensuality

Indulge in a sensual bubble bath and explore your body's luscious curves. Include your breasts and all the delicate parts of your vulva. Take your time, close your eyes, and think about the most amazing sexual and sensual experiences you had in the past and what made them so erotic for you. Masturbate if this turns you on. After your bath, dry off and look in the mirror with love and acceptance of your whole incredible body and apply a silky lotion to every part of you (except your vulva—this is a no lotion zone). Don't forget your sexy toes. Sip on something yummy and write an erotic love note to yourself, taking at least three minutes. Write out what you wish for yourself from reading this book and taking on the Sexy Challenges. Celebrate how erotic you are and how much more erotic energy you will have after each challenge.

If erotic imagining is a turn-on for you, use these same thoughts to stimulate yourself before you go to bed and join your honey. Won't he be surprised that you're all rarin' to go? I encourage you to make sensual self-exploration a part of your regular ritual. Make it a weekly routine if you really want to make your sex life a priority. The more often your inner sensuality is brought to the surface, the more easily it will come out, spill over, and infuse your life, and that of your partner, with sensual and sexual bliss.

chapter **4**

Sensational Secrets of Self-Pleasure—A Little Learning Goes a Long Way!

I change myself, I change the world. —Gloria Anzaldúa, author

Control. We women seem to have a few issues with this. Has anyone ever given you an orgasm? Please consider this question carefully. A lot of women answer yes to this when in fact, no one else has given you an orgasm—ever! Let me explain. If you have had an orgasm, it's because you *allowed* it to happen. You can be with someone who does all the "right" things, but if you aren't into him or the situation, it isn't going to happen. However, you can be with a guy who is fumbling around and doesn't really know your body, and if you are really hot for him, turned on and excited like crazy, a simple flick of a finger or tongue on your clitoris can set off an intense orgasm for you. Some women may experience orgasm from other parts of their bodies being touched if they are tuned in to their partner, turned on to the experience, and able to let go. The letting go and allowing yourself to give up control and release yourself into the experience of sexual play and pleasure is the secret to mind-blowing sex—all you have to do is allow it.

Since the clitoris is the only part of the human anatomy designed for sexual pleasure, it is our duty as women to ensure that it is used for as much sexual enjoyment as possible. Who are we to argue with God?

Celibacy is a state that many women choose. I say that you should still embrace this brilliantly crafted, natural part of you and play with it whenever possible. If you don't use it, you do lose it. The longer you go without having an orgasm, the harder it becomes for your body to remember how to do it. You can always retrain it (we are exceptional in this way), but why not keep your sexual energy flowing yourself? If you don't have someone else to play with you, do it yourself!

Get to Know Your Body

Knowledge is power, and what's better than having power over yourself? Once you learn ways to please yourself, you can more easily aid your lover to help keep you satisfied. Imagine not knowing how to ride a bike and giving one as a gift to someone with the expectation that she can ride it, only to discover she's never ridden one before either. She's seen movies of people riding bicycles, tricycles, and even unicycles, and it sure looks easy. Picture trying to teach her when all you know is how she is supposed to look on her bike as she soars down the road with the wind in her hair and a beaming smile on her face. Sure would be easier if you had a clue, wouldn't it?

Once you discover the joy your body can bring you through self-pleasure, show off for your man! Once he sees how you like to be pleased, he will have a much better idea of how to gratify you in bed. Take his hand or fingers and place them over your own for some sexy show-and-tell that will bring more intimacy into your relationship. If you sat on a bicycle, put one foot on a pedal, and balanced yourself while pushing off, it would explain how to ride much more clearly than describing those same actions. So show him and share the ways your body receives pleasure. Let the communication begin!

Developing your masturbation muscle is nourishment for your love life. Best-selling author Dr. Christiane Northrup calls it "self-cultivation." It is a way to nurture yourself and your erotic energy so you have more to offer to your relationship. Besides, you'll exude some pretty sexy vibes the more you do it. You'll be calmer, less stressed, and I'll bet you'll have a smile on your face a lot more often.

What if you don't orgasm? I think the more accurate question is, "What if you haven't had an orgasm—yet?" We can all orgasm, yet about one in ten women have not yet had the pleasure of this full letting-loose. It really comes down to you learning to unleash your inner eroticism. Figure out what honestly turns you on, accept and embrace it, and, as they said in the *Rocky Horror Picture Show*, "Give yourself over to absolute pleasure." An orgasm is simply the release of pent-up sexual tension, "release" being the key word. I hear from most women that they reach climax much faster and easier when they are alone than with their partner. This says to me that we are more easily able to let go when alone. The challenge for you, then, is to create an atmosphere in your head—or, more accurately, in your body— where you can simply *let go*! Orgasm is the peak of our sexual self-expression. As Madonna sang, "Express yourself."

Get Creative and Experiment

Some women prefer rubbing up against a pillow or stuffed animal for their pleasure. Others enjoy keeping their legs held tightly together, so you can appreciate how challenging it can be to experience orgasm during intercourse. Others like to be on their tummies, some on their backs only, and others must have their legs wide open. Your masturbatory style should be taken into account when you make love. This is useful information for your lover too!

Fantasy is a common tool men and women both use when masturbating. You can also get more advanced by slipping in some pelvic thrusting or rocking or even deep breathing. There is a masturbation practice called fire breathing that incorporates tantric techniques. I don't have room to cover these tools in this book, but you can look them up online or read Betty Dodson's book *Sex for One* (available on my Web site), a book devoted to self-pleasure!

There are many different manual masturbation techniques women use. Experiment with yourself to see how you like different strokes. The intensity of the pressure may be light or may feel like a jackhammer. We're all quite different and it may change within a lovemaking session or throughout the month depending on your hormone levels. You can squeeze your clitoris by enclosing it between both vaginal lips, pinch it quickly, rub it in circles or back and forth, or treat the clitoris like a small penis and rub along the shaft of it.

You may prefer sex toys or anything else that vibrates. Perhaps you enjoy rubbing against something with strong enough pressure to bring you to climax. Don't forget to include your nipples and other areas of your body that you may also enjoy touching both for the erotic appeal and because it feels good. As mentioned, you can add penetration when you're playing with yourself, but a lot of women focus strictly on the outside for clitoral stimulation, since more than 70 percent of us need direct clitoral stimulation to achieve orgasm.

Internally, the stronger your PC muscle (pubococcygeus), the stronger your orgasm will be, so keep it toned by doing proper Kegel exercises. You can find out more about this in my book *G-Spot PlayGuide: 7 Simple Steps to G-Spot Heaven!* available on my Web site. You can test your PC muscle strength with a free audio course at www.bladderfreedom.com.

Men Just Wanna Have Fun

Men seem to be more comfortable with the idea of masturbation than women do, but they too should enjoy some variety in their techniques. Even though he may be stimulating his penis himself, variety keeps it interesting. He can switch up the hand he uses, the speed of the stroke, the lubricant choosen, and the intensity and type of grip. He can try prolonging orgasm if he has any concerns about his orgasm being quicker than he'd like. There are stimulators for men (often called "pocket pals"; see chapter 12) that are like sleeves to insert the penis into or "gloves" with different textures; some of them even vibrate. Don't forget the other erogenous areas such as nipples, perineum, thighs, testicles, or anything else that pleases him. Again, sharing personal tricks is a wonderful way for your partner to learn what drives you wild.

Vibrators

A vibrator can greatly enhance the masturbation experience for a woman, helping her learn new ways of achieving pleasure, and can often make orgasm much easier to reach. Chapter 12 offers an overview of the wonderful world of vibrators, including types, what to look for, and how to use one. Enjoy yourself and your whole body when using a vibrator. If you've never used one before, start by using it to massage all over your body to calm and relax yourself first. Don't zero in on your clitoris right away. Think of this experience as making love to yourself. You don't want your man to go for the magic button right away, so treat yourself with the same teasing preparation. Some women enjoy penetration (inside the vagina) all by itself, and others prefer to add clitoral stimulation. Most prefer only external stimulation to get them to their pleasure peak. Whatever your preference, be sure to choose a vibrator that works for you. You'll also find more on other types of sex toys in chapter 12.

Yoko explains:

Jim and I have used sex toys together, but I usually wait until I'm alone and the kids are all out of the house so I have some privacy for using my vibrator. Since things can get tense with the strain of our new business, and my sex drive is higher than Jim's, I find it a great way to satisfy myself quickly, and I think it helps keep me more grounded. I don't spend a lot of time on other parts of my body, but I always fantasize and may read some naughty stories ahead of time to really get me in the mood. I imagine I'm in one of the scenes in the story and that helps me keep a hot picture in my mind for when I use the vibe. I often relive the same scenes over if they're really hot!

Michelle remembers back to when she masturbated a lot:

I used to be the queen of playing with myself. I was a lot hornier then. Hmm. Maybe if I started playing with myself again, my sex drive might come back.

I used to really get off on sitting up on my knees and using one hand to pump a dildo in and out while I used the other to hold a small vibrator on my clit. When I was close to coming, I would tense up my legs and, even though it was a bit awkward, I would have great orgasms.

I had one girlfriend who could only get off rubbing a bed sheet or her nightie back and forth tightly between her legs. Whatever works, I guess.

Make It a Habit

Regular sexual activity is good for you and will keep you healthy. If you aren't able to have regular sex for whatever reason, even if you are in a relationship, self-pleasure is still on the list of wonderful things to do. Not only should this be an acceptable part of your relationship, but both parties should learn that it's a much better alternative than self-neglect, building resentment, or a roving eye.

Better yet, if you can both indulge in the joys of mutual masturbation, you open up another avenue of sexual play for yourselves. Self-pleasure is an excellent option when one of you isn't in the mood. Jen discovered this with Lionel, as he has been under a lot of pressure with his business and, while her job is tiring, she doesn't bring it home with her the way Lionel does. Consequently, he is hardly ever in an amorous mood:

I've never really masturbated much. We've been together since college, and I orgasm pretty easily, so it just didn't seem necessary. I was a bit unsure when I first did it with him. I snuggled up to him in bed and his back was to me. I started rubbing my pelvis against him and he was quiet for a few minutes and I was getting more and more turned on. He asked me quietly what I wanted and I said I just wanted him to hold me close while I pleasured myself. He seemed a bit uncomfortable, but when I reassured him that I only wanted his arms wrapped around me, he sort of got into it by playing with my breasts and nuzzling my ear. It was very intimate and we seem to have more openness in our sex life that I didn't realize was missing until we got it. It's been win-win because, when he's tired, he doesn't always have his back to me anymore, so we're closer because of it.

SEXY CHALLENGE
Two to Tango

You'll Need: Lubricant and/or a vibrator (if you choose)
Prep Time: Just enough time to take a shower
Cost: $0
Raciness Factor: Bold
Benefit: Develops Intimacy and Improves Sexual Skills

Exploration is another secret to a long and satisfying sex life. Invite your sweetie to a two-session self-pleasure class for two. Take a bath or shower together to relax and so you both feel squeaky clean. Go into the bedroom and *keep the lights on* so you can watch each other. Take turns masturbating while the other watches. Enjoy the spectacle of building desire with the penis going from soft to hard and the vagina swelling and becoming wet and juicy. A blindfold may help the one who is masturbating feel a little less inhibited. Feel free to cuddle, caress each other, and whisper encouraging words to each other, but keep your eyes open so you can make mental notes of exactly what your partner is doing to bring himself such delight.

The next night, practice doing to him what you saw him doing to himself. Feel free on either night (or day) to laugh, giggle, talk, smile, joke around, and get absolutely intensely turned on! This is a brilliant exercise in building your communication skills and learning some of each others' secrets. Remember to tell him how erotic he looked and share your thoughts afterward over a glass of wine or while taking a romantic walk.

SEXY CHALLENGE
Let Me Count the Ways

You'll Need: Lubricant and/or a vibrator (if you choose)
Prep Time: None
Cost: $0
Raciness Factor: Bold
Benefit: Increases Inner Sensuality and Improves Sexual Skills

Set aside some time to experiment and play—with yourself! This time I want you to come up with three new ways to bring yourself to satisfaction. You can try using a different hand or finger(s), stimulating yourself differently (such as stimulating the left side of your clitoris instead of your usual right, or using an up-and-down motion—like with a little penis—instead of your usual circular motion), or using a toy differently (such as inside of you while you play externally with your fingers, or laying it on a pillow and "humping" or rubbing against the vibrator instead of holding it), or perhaps being in a different position than normal (such as getting up on your knees, lying on your tummy, or standing) and see how much fun you can have over a two-week period!

chapter 5

Set the Scene—Create Breathtaking Boudoirs and Other Erotic Environments

I appreciate this whole seduction thing you've got going on here, but let me give you a tip: I'm a sure thing. —**Julia Roberts,** actress, *Pretty Woman* (1990)

***Sensual* means "of** the senses," so creating sensuality in your life is simply adding all five sensory elements in pleasurable ways: lovely items to look at, scented products for arousing aromas, tasty treats to enjoy, interesting things to touch, and lovely sounds to listen to. If you can envelop yourself in sensual materials, mood lighting and music, plentiful pillows, aromatherapy, and a variety of flavors, then you will have a much more sensual life and more sex is bound to follow.

Boosting the bounce in your bedroom will come to you more easily once you have an environment that lends itself to great sex. When you have pillows that offer options for positions and the lighting and atmosphere are sensual, romance is more likely to occur naturally. If you walk into a room that is dirty, messy, and has a heap of laundry on the floor and work piled on the bedside table, who wants to make love? Change your environment to one with calming scents and a spa-like atmosphere and you will change your sex life. Guaranteed!

Location, Location, Location

Thrills can be had by simply changing the location where you make love. You can stick with the same positions you are comfortable with and change up where you make love. A new environment will heighten the thrill and make it seem like a whole new event. If you want spicy, try making love in the kitchen on the table, on the counter, or in a kitchen chair. Imagine the smile that will play along your husband's lips at breakfast the next morning as he remembers what you two were up to the night before. Make laundry more exciting by taking a tumble of your own in the soft piles of clothes on the floor. You have to wash them anyway!

Alison took this tip to heart and gave Bill a wild time in their living room after they started to get busy in the bedroom:

He started kissing me good night in bed and I knew we were going to make love, so I took his hand and he followed my naked body out into the living room. I felt him pull back a bit, but then I bent over the edge of the couch and looked over my shoulder at him. He could see my face and my back in the glow of the streetlight, and my butt was in the dark. I think that added a bit of mystery and just the right amount of naughty to make it nice for him. He's a bit shy and not too adventurous, so this was a big step for us.

You can even make your bedroom seem different by using your bed creatively. Try the same positions as usual but do them with your head at the foot of the bed or even try lying across the bed or simply switch sides so you are on his side. Try using the chair in the corner of the room or perhaps the chest at the bottom of the bed for some extra-racy fun. This is where pillows come in handy for comfort. Turn the lights on if you usually have them off, or adjust them to low. Go into your walk-in closet and give your clothes a show. Renew your lovemaking with a bit of creative flair and some slight modifications to the usual routine and make love on the bedroom floor!

Or why not revisit the memory of where you first made love? A trip down memory lane can bring back those heady feelings you had when you first started dating. Are you able to re-create the situation? Can you go to the same location or incorporate some of the same events so your sweetie recognizes the same things? Nostalgia can be a turn-on too.

$ $ $ Kim's **CASH-SAVER TIP**

Pick up a nightlight for instant mood lighting! Or go with colored lightbulbs for even sexier mood lighting. Red bulbs are the most flattering—stay away from blue or yellow.

Creating Privacy

Kids are fabulous, yet they can put a damper on romantic encounters. Sometimes you want to make love on occasions other than late at night after the kids have gone to bed. Some people have concerns about being able to fully let go if the kids are in the bedroom next door, and that will impact their lovemaking. When two people who care about each other show their emotions by making love behind closed doors, that is healthy, positive modeling for youngsters. However, if you aren't comfortable with that, have your bedroom in another area of the house or at least away from the kids' rooms. Alternatively, white-noise machines for the kids' rooms will help them sleep and will mask any other sounds, such as your moans of gratification.

Since most parents know other parents, use that as leverage. Trade off with them for date nights, afternoons, or for soccer carpooling, so you have an empty house to experiment in with your lover. You can take their kids when it's your turn and make it a fun sleepover. Everyone wins.

💜 Morning lovemaking or quickies in the middle of the night offer you variety and also provide options for kid-free fun.

Little Extras

Freshen up the romance factor of your whole house. You can revitalize your love life by creating sexy nooks and little stashes of romantic finds so when the mood strikes you for love, you'll be ready. Find some small drawstring bags of velvet or some other sensuous material and pop in two or three of the following simple and sexy accessories for a hot time. Tuck them away in a kitchen cupboard, down in the family room, or in the spare room or den. Just don't forget they're there!

- ⊙ Condoms (flavored for fun)
- ⊙ Flavored lubricant pillow packs (one-time use packs)
- ⊙ Breath freshener
- ⊙ Red lipstick (so you can turn on instant sex appeal)
- ⊙ Flavored lip gloss

- Mini vibrator or other sex toy
- Small bottles of massage oil
- Handcuffs (for the adventurous)
- Blindfolds
- Vibrating penis rings (for the bold)

Look at your home through the eyes of a lover. There must be a few spots that are begging for two lovers to cavort and play. Like Alison and Bill, do you have a couch that is perfect for bending over? Here are some spots to give you some ideas:

- A recliner
- A furry rug in front of the fireplace
- The stairs, with pillows from the couch
- A sturdy desk
- The bathroom counter
- A private back patio deck
- The shower (see chapter 15 for more)
- A window seat
- A chair in the foyer
- The guest bedroom

Recipe for Lovemaking

Ingredients for love are often found in the kitchen. Rustle up some kitchen treats such as ice cubes, a spoon, towels for comfort, fresh fruit, chocolate spread or whipped cream, an electric carving knife with no blade (okay, this is pretty racy, but it makes a great vibrator in a pinch!), and you can have a pretty daring and erotic time. Marcia got brave and used the steamy kitchen food scene from *9½ Weeks* as her inspiration:

Don and I have never really been that adventurous in bed and I often fake my orgasm to keep him happy. He works hard and I don't like making him work hard in bed too. The kids were out at my mom's for the night and I put on a lacy bra and panty set (which turned me on) with a nice robe over them and had dinner ready for Don when he got home from work. We each had a glass of wine with dinner to relax us both, and I worked up my nerve to ask him if he wanted to see what was under my robe for dessert.

I was really nervous, but I could feel myself getting wetter as he followed me to the fridge. We'd seen the movie years ago and I was hoping he'd remember it. The lights had already been dimmed because we ate by candlelight. I opened the fridge door and dropped my robe as I turned to face him. His mouth dropped open and I thought it would hit the floor. I had a bowl of cut-up fruit, ice cubes, whipped cream, and some chocolate syrup the kids used, all within reach. I pretended I was Kim Basinger and put a towel from the counter on the floor in front of the fridge and kneeled down in front of my husband. I won't say what happened next, but we fed each other the fruit with the syrup and whipped cream and had the hottest sex I can remember, and I didn't have to fake it!

Taking Your Love Public

Some adventurous couples find that the thrill of getting caught is enticing. It excites them because of the potential danger. You don't really want to get caught, though, so be safe. If you have a nice tall fence in your backyard, use it as a shield to cover your outdoor love-fest. The beach is always a treat, as long as you have a blanket to protect you from the sand. Your car can be romantic, but only if you have lots of room. The backseat tends to be more spacious and can bring back hot memories of making out when you were younger. A secluded area in a park can be very romantic, but have a blanket handy (keep one in the trunk of your car) just in case someone comes along.

No Boundaries

Traveling? Try this when you are away to help make a boring hotel room a little more ready for romance: spritz a little of your favorite scent or perfume into the air of a hotel room or on the pillows on your bed. Spray some essential oil or place a few drops on a cotton ball and tuck it into your pillow to keep your senses tuned in for love. The essences of patchouli, neroli, and rose are reported to be wonderful for stimulating arousing thoughts. If your man is on the road, try a quick, light spritz of your favorite scent in his briefcase. Smell is the sense most strongly connected to memory. He'll think of you every time he opens it, as the aroma gently wafts up to tickle his nose.

Another thing you can do to help remind him of you while he is away is to tuck a sultry photo of yourself somewhere he is sure to find it. Alternatively, you can e-mail it to him. Men are typically very visual, so this reminder is sure to be remembered and to keep him stoked for you until he gets home!

One more sexy travel tip for you. Just as pregnant women keep a bag ready at all times, women who are serious about their love lives should too. Be prepared for those spur-of-the-moment trips so you aren't caught short and wanting (translation: frustrated). Use this checklist for the necessities of a sexy travel cache:

- Massage oil
- Condoms or other birth control
- Lubricant (I always recommend flavored)
- A sex toy or two
- Your sexiest pair of heels
- Batteries (It's not fun to have your toy stop at just the wrong moment!)
- A feather
- A scarf
- Lingerie
- Garters
- Stick-on tattoos
- Lipstick (for your lips, or to leave naughty messages on napkins)

What else can you think of that would be a perfectly decadent surprise for your man? Go ahead and list a few more items that you know your guy would enjoy:

_____

_____

_____

Don't be intimidated at the thought of introducing accessories to your boudoir, packing naughty surprises for your sexy travel bag, or adding to the secret stashes stored around your house. Always keep your eyes open for romantic finds such as scarves, high heels, scented candles and their holders, sexy lampshades, gorgeous floor or wall coverings, comfy pillows, peacock feathers, and other delights at discount stores, outlets, or among castoffs from friends. Keep a list handy in your purse of the items you are looking for so when you spot a yard sale or bargain shop, you don't wander aimlessly. Remember the idea of setting your intention for hot romance. Keeping the idea in front of you will help you see things in a different light and you will more easily appreciate their multiuse appeal.

SEXY CHALLENGE
Romantic Renovation

You'll Need: Sensual materials, flowers in a vase (fresh preferred), scented candles
Prep Time: None—just do it
Cost: $0+
Raciness Factor: Regular
Benefit: Develops Intimacy

Create a relaxing and sensual boudoir environment and celebrate by making love in a new room—yours!

A cluttered room does *not* promote romance. Remove these items from the bedroom:

- All laundry
- All piles of papers
- All books (except this and other sexy ones)
- Anything work related
- Any clutter

Hide these items in another room, a hamper, a closet, or a box if necessary. Cover a box with a sexy sheet of satin, silk, or an animal-print robe you may not have used in a while. Put a vase of flowers on top and perhaps a bottle of massage oil or, better yet, a candle that you can melt to use as massage oil (purchase from my Web site). Ah, serenity. Pick at least five of the following (or create some of your own):

- Remove the TV (unless you're using it for sexy movies) or cover it with another lovely piece of material.
- Find a lovely piece of art for the walls that makes you feel sensual. Kid's art or photos of grandparents are not conducive to hot romance. Give them a place of honor elsewhere.
- Add scented candles, potpourri, or flowers to the bedside table.
- Get a dimmer switch for the overhead light, add a low wattage lamp, or try a nightlight.
- Bring erotica, adult movies, condoms, sex toys, scarves, oils, lubes, or lotions within easy reach.
- Have a radio or iPod for mood music.
- Keep this book (and other sexy books) in a drawer, under your mattress, or on the bedside table.
- Put your best sheets and lots of pillows on the bed!

$ $ $ Kim's **CASH-SAVER TIP**

Pick up scented candles, potpourri, or air fresheners from a dollar store.

Look in your basement, linen closet, or thrift store for sensual slipcover materials or wall art. Paint walls a new color that helps you feel sensual (mis-tints from a paint store are cheap!) Or place a few mirrors around so you can enjoy catching a glimpse of you and your lover entangled in each other's arms.

chapter **6**

chapter **6**

Kissing Your Way to the Top—From Kindling to Kinky, Never-Fail Techniques

You should be kissed and often by someone who knows how.
—Clark Gable, actor, *Gone with the Wind* (1939)

If you want an easy way to set your man on fire, develop your repertoire of kisses. This chapter is chock-full of simple, sexy, and sultry kisses for you to practice on someone very, very lucky. Wet those lips and get smooching!

Look, Lick, and Lock Lips

- Tease him with your eyes. Lick your lips seductively and move in toward him one step at a time, ever so slowly, to tease him even further. Let the energy spark between you. You can see the sheen of perspiration on his upper lip. Yes, you're close enough to feel his hot breath on your cheeks as you twist your head slightly. Bypass his mouth and softly brush your lips against his cheek. Rest your hand over his heart and whisper into his ear that you can feel his heart beating. Ask if he can feel it too. Run your other hand down his back and grab his butt cheek, squeezing just enough so he knows you mean it. Then pull him to you and plant a hard, wet kiss on his lips for three or four seconds. Pull away abruptly, whisper for him to have a nice day. Turn and go back to what you were doing.

○ High heels are a great way to improve your kissing. Women tend to feel more confident in something that helps them feel sexy. Confidence is the number one aphrodisiac, so any way you can find to add some is a bonus. Besides, a few extra inches can give you a feeling of greater power, which will infuse your kisses. You can add stockings to the high heels and maybe nothing else but a garter and smile to really heat things up.

❤ Learning to push both your boundaries and your partner's will continue to add depth and dimension to your love life. Kissing is a simple, fun, and pretty risk-free way to start.

Tie, Touch, and Torture Him with Kisses

○ Grab a scarf or his tie (undo the knot) and slowly wrap it around his eyes like a blindfold. Strip him down slowly and silently and practice kissing him over his whole body. The blindfold ensures he won't know where your next kiss will land, so take your time drawing out the anticipation. You should soon see the results of your efforts in his growing erection. You can strip yourself down as well and use your whole body while you plant kisses on him from his forehead to his toes. Touch is said to boost your immune system, so consider this a great way to keep the doctor away. Be seductive, don't hurry through this, and enjoy every second!

- Wandering hands help you learn to give a full body kiss, since it seems natural for the rest of your body to follow the lead of your hands. Thinking can throw you off, so let go and imagine your whole body is able to show your honey how much you want to kiss him all over every delicious inch. Focus on one area at a time, such as the torso, and take your time there. Wrap yourself around his legs while you plant a hundred torso kisses. Then move along to kissing his legs. While you do that, use your hands and your legs to rub up against him. Some of these areas are more easily kissed if you're both lying down.

Take no prisoners! Well, okay, maybe just one. Alison discovered the next technique works well if you lean your partner up against a wall:

> I was feeling particularly randy one night and got home to find Bill had already arrived and was standing in the kitchen, loosening his tie and enjoying a drink. I didn't say anything, but walked over, put his drink on the counter, and leaned him back against the wall beside the fridge.

I grabbed his wrists and lifted his arms above his head. I held them there with one hand while the other roamed over his body, caressing his chest and squeezing his butt cheeks (he has a tremendous butt!). I kissed him with all the passion I was feeling. As my intensity increased, I kissed him harder and deeper while paying attention to whether he was pulling back or not. I had to pay a bit of attention to his lips and body so I didn't freak him out by going too hard, too fast. I slowly made my way down to the front of his pants with my free hand and was surprised and impressed by the firmness of his erection. That got me even hotter. I've been trying to find out what makes his inner animal tick, and this seemed to be working! I really enjoyed taking charge and have to say, for the first time in a while, I didn't hear one word about how his day went.

This scenario can be especially powerful if you aren't usually the one who initiates lovemaking.

Regular attention to the 10-Second Kiss will do wonders for a ho-hum sex life. The trick is to be fully 100 percent present for all ten seconds (or longer if it goes that way). What I mean is not to be thinking of shopping, the kids, or even wondering what he's thinking about. You don't want to think, you want to *feel* the 10-Second Kiss. Spontaneity also helps add to the mystique of it all. So what is it? Quite simply, it is ten whole seconds of true, solid, full attention to kissing your partner. It may be soft, hard, slow, or fast, as long as it lasts for at least ten seconds. There is even a book written about it called *The 10 Second Kiss* by Ellen Kreidman that you can check out at www.kimswitnicki .com/greatsexforhardtimes.

10-Second Bliss

You'll Need: Your lips and his
Prep Time: None
Cost: $0
Raciness Factor: Regular
Benefit: Improves Sexual Skills

This will keep a spring in your step and will help you feel sexy all day long. Practice the 10-Second Kiss for ten days at ten different times of day or using ten different techniques or tongue strokes.

Michelle shocked Dave when she tried the 10-Second Kiss on him out of the blue:

> *It's been so long since we've really kissed with any passion that he didn't know what to do with himself other than respond back. It took him a few of those seconds to fully participate, but when he did, I got a bit of a flutter in my tummy. You have no idea what that did for me. I felt myself getting a little emotional, so I stopped. But I know Dave felt something too. After I stopped, I just opened my eyes, looked at him intently, and kissed him quick like usual and then went back to doing my dishes. He hasn't brought it up, but I'm hoping he is looking forward to it happening again!*

After any kiss, as you're walking away, do a quick double-back and plant another one on him just for fun!

In the Moment

Reward yourself by being fully present and in the moment, not only for all of your kissing, but also for any intimate activity. One of the secrets my clients discover about themselves is that a great sex life is not about what they are *doing* but who they are *being* when they do it. Being present is a habit that will reward you in all areas of your life, but with lovemaking, it is the magic ingredient that makes *all* the difference.

Make Time for What Matters

The tongue and the lips are the two main body parts you use for applying great kissing. Where they go is totally up to you! The other tool required is creative abandon. Take your time. When we were young, a lot of us enjoyed making out for hours. It's a great prelude to sex and can also be a main event! When we've been in a longer-term relationship, the kissing tends to get very matter of fact, peck on the cheek, and dry as cardboard. Let's change that. Kissing is a very quick and simple way to add spice, so sprinkle some magic kissing dust over your man or buy a sprig of plastic mistletoe at your local crafts shop and take a minute here or there to show him how much you desire him; your desire is bound to rise too.

When you go to bed tonight, ask for a good night kiss and really make it count. Pretend you are back in school or whenever kissing was the high point of your day. If he doesn't respond at first, murmur or moan how wonderful it is to have his lips on yours. Encourage him and keep on kissing him until he gets that you are serious. Let him know you'd like to make a habit of kissing him good night to wrap up your day, so he knows it isn't an automatic prelude to sex. It is simply a way to show appreciation for all he does, show him how much he means to you, and keep your erotic energy flowing. Bon appétit!

Kissing Do's:
- Do keep things slippery.
- Do send your tongue on an exploratory mission. Feel under his lips, along his teeth, and over other parts of his face too.
- Do keep your breath smelling fresh and kissable.
- Do use your hands to expand the experience, caressing the face, neck, ears, etc.

Kissing Don'ts:
- Don't apply too much pressure, especially if your partner is pulling away.
- Don't be a wimp with pressure so he barely feels your lips, unless you are deliberately teasing him with the promise of more to come.
- Don't slobber. Use saliva for keeping things slippery, not soggy.
- Don't attempt to put your tongue down your partner's throat.
- Don't limit yourself to the face. The skin is a huge amusement park. Travel around this exciting erogenous zone using your tongue and lips as wonderful instruments of pleasure.

●●● Kim's **QUICKIE TIP**

Having a beverage handy (even a bottle of water) during a kissing-fest is a must to keep your mouth juicy! Try melting an ice cube in your mouth for cool fun, or sparkling juice to keep his taste buds tingling as his tongue meets yours. . . .

Slurp, suck, and *lick*: what yummy words they are. We usually associate them with desserts such as ice cream and Popsicles. Marcia decided to use the time she spends at home with the kids to do some training for an imaginary kissing Olympics. Her special practice started with ice cubes:

> *I'm determined to get more from my sex life, so I undertook some serious preparation. I never really saw the big deal about making out and figured I was a lousy kisser, so I started sucking on ice cubes and practiced flipping them around in my mouth using my tongue to maneuver them about. I sometimes would bore a hole almost through the ice cube with the tip of my tongue melting it. When I got good at that, I graduated to Popsicles: the big, fat, round ones. Pretty soon I could eat a whole one without really using my teeth at all. I mostly used my tongue to lick it. I'm sure this has helped my oral sex confidence too!*
>
> *Finally I indulged in a lot of fruit cocktail so I could practice separating the little pieces from one another inside my mouth. I don't know how much my kissing skills actually improved, but I feel like a kissing champion now, and Don gets a lot more good night kisses, which sometimes even lead to great sex.*

Mix it up and employ a little variety with your tongue strokes. Try some light, teasing, and short strokes with maybe a little nibble at the end. Then try out quick flicks and some long strokes. More delicate spots on the body such as the inner elbow or behind the knee may not respond well to love bites, but experiment with your lover to see what he likes best. Tender bites and gentle nibbling are most appropriate to test out on areas where you have bigger muscles or more fatty tissue such as the legs, buttocks, and arms. You can also run your teeth along the skin for yet another sensation. Have fun!

●●● Kim's **QUICKIE TIP**

As we become more aroused, our sensitivity to pain decreases, so we can handle more intense sensations the more turned on we are!

Recipe for Delicious Kisses

Delicious-tasting lips and mouths are very inviting and arousing. Try the recipe below for some steamy kissing. Making out will make you hunger for more to come with the following elixir to spritz into your mouth fresh from a perfume atomizer or to discreetly swig from a jar or glass. Use it after eating a romantic meal to get dessert started early.

- 1 teaspoon fresh mint leaves
- 1 teaspoon rosemary leaves
- 1 teaspoon anise or fennel seeds
- Zest from one orange
- 2 cups spring water

Mix all ingredients and bring gently to a boil. Simmer for fifteen to twenty minutes. Cool your potion, strain it, and store the infusion for up to a week in a sealed or covered jar in the refrigerator. Shake before using. Take one tablespoon each time and swish it around your mouth completely.

Or . . .

If you're in a real hurry, mix a teaspoon of baking soda into an eight-ounce glass of water and add a drop of pure peppermint oil. Minty fresh and kissable in a flash. Imagine your lover's surprise when you let him know you made this delicious kissing potion yourself. It will tell him without words how much you love making out with him!

$ $ $ Kim's **CASH-SAVER TIP**

Pick up flavored ChapStick or lip gloss at the drugstore for quick and easy make-out fun.

💜 Kissing is a great workout! You use thirty-four muscles when you kiss. . . . Now, how can you build this into *your* exercise routine?

SEXY CHALLENGE
Three's a Charm

You'll Need: Your lips and his willing body
Prep Time: None
Cost: $0

Raciness Factor: Bold
Benefit: Improves Sexual Skills

Use your imagination and think of areas on your man that are often ignored but that he might like some extra attention paid to. Blow his mind by picking three body parts you don't usually kiss and ravishing them with your lips, tongue, and teeth for at least five minutes each before bringing your hands or any of your other body parts into the fun!

SEXY CHALLENGE
Good Night Kiss

You'll Need: His lips and your willing body
Prep Time: None
Cost: $0
Raciness Factor: Bold
Benefit: Improves Sexual Skills, Develops Intimacy

Next time you are in bed together and your sweetie isn't exhausted, ask him if he would do something for you. Let him know how much you love his lips and describe how it feels when they are on your body. Tell him what it is about his lips that makes you lust after him. Then ask him sweetly if he would kiss your _____ (pick a favorite kissable body part) for thirty seconds to help you fall into a dreamy sleep. See what happens from there!

chapter **7**

Rev Your Sexual Engine into High Gear with Simple Sex-Drive Boosters

Sex without love is merely healthy exercise.
—**Robert A. Heinlein, science-fiction writer**

Low libido (sex drive) is one of the most common concerns for the women I speak with. When men come up to me at events or call me on the phone, their most common questions involve their partners' low libidos. There are so many different factors impacting your body's ability to have a strong, healthy sex drive. Some of them are:

- Stress (about money, kids, work, life)
- Fatigue
- Feeling overwhelmed
- Hormone levels
- Ill health
- Emotional concerns

- Relationship issues
- Seasonal Affective Disorder

Some of these, such as stress, fatigue, and feeling over-whelmed, can be greatly affected by implementing some lifestyle changes such as de-stressing with more sex and increasing physical exercise to combat fatigue. While the solutions may seem at odds with the problem, they really do work. Other issues such as hormones, health, and emotional concerns may need the intervention of a professional to help you sort out medications and start to take better care of yourself. Bad weather may impact how you feel, which can affect your libido. If it is a huge problem, you might consider moving to a climate better suited to your needs.

Try my M.E.D.S. plan at the end of this chapter for some inexpensive and safe ways to boost your libido naturally. Is there simply a magic pill to help your sex life? Sadly, no. However, some herbal supplements may improve specific health issues (such as poor blood circulation), which can certainly impact your sex life overall. Life is too short to spend it not having great sex!

First Step

Reassure yourself first by getting a thorough checkup by your doctor. Many of the most common drugs have a negative impact on the libido. If your hormone levels are wonky, a cream, a supplement, or a few hormone shots may be suggested by your doctor or naturopath to fix you right up.

Talk Is Key

Communication is crucial if you find your sex drive diminishing. Bring up the subject with your partner so he knows you still love and desire him but your body isn't cooperating as you would like. He may be thinking you're losing interest in him, so don't be surprised at the sense of relief he expresses when you share what's been happening for you. Before we get to some of the simple treatments for low sex drive, I'd like to offer some solutions for how you can handle the situation in your relationship.

Maintain Intimacy

Just because you aren't having a lot of sex doesn't mean you should lose intimacy. Whether there are health challenges restricting your ability to make love, your sex drive is low due to medications, you are too tired, or you simply can't fit it in right now, it is important for your relationship to maintain or rebuild your authentic connection. If you let a lack of sex create a lack of intimacy, romance, and connection, you will feel a gap in your closeness that may get wider and wider if it isn't addressed head on. Juanita and Carlos never had much of a sex life, and she has never felt fully satisfied. She decided to take the bull by the horns since, at forty-five, she doesn't want to waste any more time. Juanita started with the basics to gain more intimacy, and hopefully to set off some sparks and relight their love flame. This is how she rebuilt their bond:

> With two kids in the house, it's hard to find places for romance, so I started inviting Carlos into the shower with me. The kids used to roll their eyes and smirk, but they're

getting used to it. I like that we can have special time for us while still being available if the kids need us for an emergency.

We started by washing each others' backs, and now he'll wash my hair and sometimes even shave my legs. When we started out, I would wrap a big bath towel around him when we got out and sometimes I'd comb his hair. Now, after the shower he wraps me in the towel and pats me dry. He puts lotion all over me and makes me feel like a princess.

There isn't any sex attached, so it's all totally relaxing and comfortable. We laugh and entertain each other for the sheer fun of it. I love how I'm feeling with him now. I touch him and show affection much more and am noticing that I have more interest in exploring my sexuality.

Two Rules

The mind–body connection is an intensely powerful one. It's important that you never do anything sexually with your body that you aren't 100 percent into doing—especially penetration. Your body will remember if you do anything uncomfortable, and you can set up a negative cycle in which your body tightens up and won't allow anything (toy, finger, or penis) inside of you. This results in painful intercourse. This condition can be remedied, but my suggestion is to simply prevent it instead. Plus, you can end up building resentments against your partner. So stick to only doing things that you agree to.

My Definition of Healthy Sexuality:
- 100 percent consensual for all parties involved
- 100 percent pleasurable for all parties involved

As long as everyone is having consensual sex, whether it's just you or you're with five of your friends, it's all good. Everyone experiences pleasure differently, so as long as you are all feeling good, then go for it!

How to Handle It

Honesty is another great libido booster, if only for the weight it can lift from you, thereby freeing you up to actually get turned on. Share gently when you aren't in the mood for love and be okay with it. Be willing to cuddle your sweetie as he masturbates, or be okay with reading your book while he indulges in self-pleasure. Once you can do this with comfort and grace, you may find that the motion or sound of your lover arousing himself gets you turned on. If you are angry, resentful, or anxious, there won't be room for you to get turned on. Practice saying, "No thanks" in ways that are okay for both of you.

Checking In

I'm not an advocate of having sex because it is your duty or because you want to do it as a favor to your lover. However, I do believe you can make love in a healthy way even if you don't start out in the mood.

If your lover makes motions that he wants to make love and you're tired or aren't feeling well, take a moment to check in and see how you're really feeling. Even if you aren't turned on, notice if you *wish you felt more desire*. Often, if you go through the motions, you will start to get aroused eventually. If you really would like to have some connection with your partner, check in with yourself to make sure you absolutely, 100 percent would like to have this desire be stronger. If your *willingness* is 100 percent, then you are still consenting, even if you aren't turned on yet but know it will come. The worst thing is to be grumbling under your breath or in your head that you're only doing this because he's your husband and you should. You need to want to do it.

Jen started checking in with herself on the odd occasion when Lionel wanted sex and she didn't:

> *He would mostly put the moves on me the night before he was heading out of town for a week to see a client. Usually I stay up late helping him pack and prepare, so I'm pretty beat by the time we hit the sheets. I used to give in and have sex with him, but on those occasions I wouldn't climax, and I usually do quite easily. I think I was too busy feeling frustrated.*
>
> *Now I check in, and if I really don't want to have sex, I let him know, and he's okay with that and we just go to sleep. More often, though, when I really think about it, instead of reacting, I realize that even though I'm tired, I think it's sweet that he wants to make love, even though he is probably tired too. I really miss him while he's gone, so it is really great to have a quick shot of sex before he leaves. Once my mind shifts, it really doesn't take me that long to get into it, and those times I do have great orgasms!*

Turn Yourself On

We check in now with Michelle, who was going to try masturbating again to get her juices and her sexual energy flowing:

The first few times I tried masturbating again I used my own fingers the way I used to do, and all I got was frustrated. Maybe I was trying too hard, but it just didn't seem to be happening for me. Then I dug out a vibrator that a friend had given me as a gag gift. This time I had a bath and did some fantasizing the way Kim suggested. Well, I got turned on and went to bed with my toy. Frank was out with the boys, so I had some time to myself.

I had a small tube of lubricant that I used to get the vibrator wet, and I put a bit on my clit too. Since I was alone, I didn't feel bad that I was still dry. I started the vibe on a low speed to get used to the feeling again. It didn't take long until I was enjoying the feeling quite a lot, and I was right back into my fantasy from the bath. I started breathing heavier and getting really warm. I started grinding myself into the toy and was imagining it was the lusty lover from my fantasy whose head was between my legs, licking me like crazy. I started rocking my pelvis back and forth, building up the intensity. I increased the speed on the vibrator and whoa! I went from having a pretty good time to having an awesome time. It only took a few more seconds from there, and I exploded with my first orgasm in about three years! I rocked back and forth like a madwoman, feeling my own juices dribbling out of me. It was amazing. There is hope!

💜 Develop your orgasmic ability and your capacity for orgasm will increase. The more orgasms you have, the easier it will be to have more orgasms!

How to Help Him

Testosterone levels (partially responsible for the sex drive) fluc-
tuate for men during a twenty-four hour period. Levels are high-
est in the morning, which is why men typically have a beautiful
erection first thing when they wake up. Testosterone levels also
cause approximately seven erections each night for the average
man. If your man is having issues with not being able to achieve
or maintain his erection due to stress, consider the following
option if you typically journey to the bathroom in the middle of
the night to urinate. Instead of going back to bed and right to
sleep, why not reach out to your man and see if his penis is hard?
If not, you can always gently try to help it along. A bit of help
from you and a stress-free environment (he's likely calm when
sleeping), and your trip to the bathroom can result in a quickie
ending with both of you smiling.

This also works if you're just too tired during the day or
before bed. If your libido is drawn to it, why not take advantage
of the variety offered by some early-morning delight?

M.E.D.S. Plan

As mentioned at the start of this chapter, here is my M.E.D.S.
plan for helping you safely, naturally, and economically pump
up your libido. The secret is to maintain a healthy body and
attitude.

M Is for Mind-set

Imagine yourself wearing your worn but comfy woolies—how
sexy do you feel? You might feel warm and fuzzy, but it's hard to
really feel like a sultry vixen in flannel. How do you feel when

you wear silky lingerie? What about a beautiful corset or black stockings under your clothes with pair of high heels? What else makes you *feel* like a hot mama? Sexy is a state of mind. If you want to ooze sexy and sensuality, you can! Simply deciding that you will put time and attention into your sex life will do wonders for increasing your desire. The act or intention of choosing to want more will draw sexy things to you. You get more of what you focus on in life, so instead of thinking about how awful your sex life is, keep thinking about all the wonderful parts of it and how much more incredible it is becoming.

Inattention to your sexuality will rob you of your youth quickly, since your vitality will lessen, your life force will become more fragile, and your immune system will weaken. If you pump up your love life, your ecstasy will keep you strong, vital, and young!

BONUS

If you want help connecting with your sexiness on a regular basis, download my audio coaching process to help you get a head start on feeling sultry whenever you want to. My gift to you, this process is called the Sacred Sexy Circle. Go to the special page on my Web site (www.kimswitnicki .com/greatsexforhardtimes) created just for you to download it for free!

E Is for Exercise

One of the main reasons for being fit is to be sexy! Accept the incentive! Being fit brings confidence, which is the number one aphrodisiac. Having sex is great aerobic exercise. If you're tired and out of shape, you are less likely to want to have sex. When you're overweight, you are also more tired and may have body-image issues, which can mean you're less inclined to make love. Losing extra pounds is also at the top of most lists on how to cure snoring. So slimming down can help some couples return to sleeping in the same bed if they have been apart due to one person's snoring. You're likely to have more sex if you sleep in the same bed. Sex also keeps stress, tension, and depression at bay, so you'll end up having more sex if you simply have more sex.

●●● Kim's **QUICKIE TIP**

Get moving! Go rock climbing, dancing, power walking, golfing, or swimming, play squash or lawn bowling, or go workout together. When you both move and sweat together, your endorphins will be up for both of you, so you never know what else may rise. I was speaking of your temperature (wink, wink).

D Is for Diet (Including Water)

This may not sound sexy, but a diet rich in fruits, vegetables, and lean protein will keep your organs in peak condition for lovemaking, according to the National College of Natural Medicine. When low in energy, head for the bedroom not the fridge!

Chinese medicine says that sexual energy or *chi* is in our kidneys, so keep them strong and healthy. Some ways to do this include eating:

- beef
- blueberries
- celery
- dark mushrooms
- eggs
- lamb
- lobster
- miso
- molasses in warm water
- mussels
- ocean fish
- olives
- oysters
- shrimp
- walnuts
- well-cooked tofu

Don't eat fried foods, creams, excess sugar, salt, saturated fat, or highly processed foods. These make it harder for you to reach orgasm. Tobacco, alcohol, and coffee leach nutrients from your body and dampen desire! Doesn't that give you *even more* incentive to change habits you know are bad for you?

Stay hydrated. You can survive for three weeks with no food but only for three to four days with no water. We're 90 percent water, so it is obviously critical to your health. Alcohol numbs nerve endings, decreases lubrication, and can depress libido, so try water instead. Staying hydrated also provides something to sweat off in bed!

●●● Kim's QUICKIE TIP

Phenylethylamine is the magic ingredient in chocolate that raises endorphins (natural antidepressants) so we feel good after eating chocolate, as long as we don't eat too much. Go for wholesome and yummy dark, organic chocolate.

S Is for Sleep

Relaxation and rest are essential to good health. Making love helps you relax and get to sleep, as the endorphins released will help calm you. Your habits and sleeping environment deeply affect your ability to relax and sleep, so look around your bedroom! Read chapter 5 to create a sensual boudoir that will induce romance. A good night's sleep is like going for a free beauty treatment. When your body is at rest, it heals, recuperates, builds, repairs, and even removes fluids from the skin so we glow youthfully.

Get hugs throughout your day to keep you relaxed. Snuggle and kiss before sleeping. Practice doing it with "No sex" as the rule—one that can be
broken!

Simply taking some easy steps, such as drinking and eating
better, getting more rest, exercising, and thinking more positively, can give you immediate results in your sex life—even if it
is good already! If you choose to say no to implementing *any* of
these changes, what are you really saying yes to? If you don't
make *any* changes at all, what will your love life look like in a
month? In six months? In a year? You are in control of your own
choices. Go for what will give you the greatest satisfaction.

SEXY CHALLENGE
Let's Play, Honey!

You'll Need: You and him naked
Prep Time: None
Cost: $0
Raciness Factor: Bold
Benefit: Develops Intimacy

Snuggle together naked and kiss each other good night for two
solid weeks of eroticism without having intercourse. No sex for
two weeks. You can caress and rub and massage but no genital
stimulation of your partner. Once you let go of the pressure,
you'll be amazed at how much better you feel about the idea of
sex! You can engage in self-pleasure (which is the only sex you
can have during this time) if you get really turned on while cud-
dling, but you have to be together any time you masturbate

during the two weeks. Commit that you will let each other know (a sexy e-mail, text, or phone call) with a secret code word that lets your partner know when you want to play with yourself, and make time to be together to experience the fun of being with your lover for this sensual play.

Bonus points if you schedule one fun exercise activity to do together each week to get your heart rate up. Enjoy!

chapter **8**

Talking Flirty to Talking Dirty— Communication Is Your Key to Scorching Sex

The most important marriage skill is listening to your partner in a way that they can't possibly doubt that you love them. **—Diane Sollee, marriage counselor**

Communication is the single most important factor affecting sexual satisfaction. Virtually any sexual concerns or troubles can be helped and even corrected by talking about them with your lover. Once you develop more comfort with your own sexuality, it becomes easier to chat about it. Openness and trust can be difficult with something as sensitive and core to our identities as our sexuality. Once you break through that and recognize your vulnerability, even with someone you love, huge progress can be made. If you can talk comfortably about sex, you can talk about money, parenting, or anything! Let me share some of the secrets of powerful talk in the bedroom as well as how to approach the subject outside of the bedroom so you can have your best sex ever.

Lots of women deprive themselves of immense satisfaction by placing their partners' egos or pleasure before their own. This is not the way to sexual bliss! Would you want your man to swallow his feelings, bypass his own pleasure, and make assumptions about what is best for you without sharing that information with you? I invite you to try asking for what you want and to discover how incredible it is when you receive it. The number one priority men report to me is ensuring that their partner is satisfied. Your man wants to please you!

Too often we have hang-ups—because of upbringing, religious beliefs, or our society—about what is "good" or proper sexual behavior. These inhibitions limit our ability to expand, explore, and thereby enhance our lovemaking. Remember my definition of healthy sexuality:

- 100 percent consensual for all parties involved
- 100 percent pleasurable for all parties involved

Take the Lead

Lots of men secretly (or obviously) like a woman who takes charge in bed. This is a huge generalization, since there are women who like a man who is in control. Typically we sexually yearn for the opposite of what is happening in our everyday life. We don't want it full-time, but it can be an erotically charged evening when a usually submissive woman decides to take over and be the sexual aggressor. Yoko plays with this scenario on occasion and wanted to step it up a little by adding some sexy talk with Jim. Here is what she did:

Every now and then I take control and become more aggressive in the bedroom. I want to keep making things interesting for both of us. We only blended our families together two years ago but we've been in business together (and dating) for nearly five years. I think it's important to keep our love life spicy.

Jim is pretty masculine, so it really turns me on when he lets me take over. Last time I had him tied to the bedposts, he was squirming and writhing around and his body told me he was pretty turned on. I totally love hearing him moan, and I usually tease him and lick his body all over and then bring him to orgasm with my mouth. With him being in that submissive place, I can be a bit more aggressive than normal. This time I went even further.

I used a gorgeous silk scarf I had and used it to cover up his eyes. I tied it tightly behind his head. My heart was beating a little faster, and it really added another layer of submission, which made me feel a little braver. Then I started whispering things in his ear and asking him questions.

"Do you like being tied up?"

"Does it get you hot when I do this?"

"What would you like me to do next?"

"Do you want this harder?"

I started asking the questions louder and stronger, building my confidence with every answer he gave me. I was surprised by a few of his answers, like when I was pinching his nipple and he wanted me to do it harder and harder. I had no idea that he liked that. Frankly, I don't think he even knew! Adding the blindfold gave me the

confidence to ask, and having that dialogue while we were
in bed in the heat of passion in that way just opened things
up for us. I can't wait to have him try it on me!

●●● Kim's **QUICKIE TIP**

Each night this week, practice feeling turned on, being more assertive, or seducing your honey before walking into your bedroom and see what happens.

Since talking is crucial to learning and exploring together, let's look at how else we communicate. Experts say that 65 to 90 percent of our communication is body language. So how do you pass along messages with your eyes, limbs, and general body moves? Women are naturally good at flirting. We can bat our eyelashes, tilt our heads down while looking up seductively, or simply wink at the cute guy across the room. These are usually deliberate moves. What we often miss are the subtle things we do unconsciously that signal either "Come closer" or "Get lost!"

Develop your ability to recognize how you're holding your body and presenting yourself. Be aware that others may make assumptions about your body language thinking you are flirting or feeling frisky when you are simply scratching an itch or batting away a bug. Whatever your signals are, learn how they are being interpreted by having a conversation with your partner to see if what you are putting out is what he is picking up.

If you stand with your arms crossed or turned away from your man, roll your eyes, or watch TV when he speaks, he will pick up that you aren't being open and accepting of him. If you face him, tilt your head his way, lean forward if sitting or have an open posture if standing, he'll likely be more receptive to you. Your tone of voice will also say a lot, underscoring your words.

When you gently touch his knee or arm while speaking, it shows sincerity and a desire to be closer. Combine this with looking into his eyes and you're more likely to connect when broaching the sensitive subject of sex. The direct physical contact of touching while speaking or listening is also useful for emphasis. The healing properties of touch have long been proven beneficial to humans.

The Power of Eye Contact

The intensity of eye gazing can be a powerful aphrodisiac if you do it with someone you love. Get into a very comfortable position sitting across from each other with your faces twelve to eighteen inches apart. You can do a more advanced version, if you like, by sitting really close together and match your breathing. Pick one eye (for example, your right and his left) and gaze into it lovingly for five to fifteen minutes. You may giggle at first, but it will pass. Enjoy the erotic energy you bring between you.

Understanding Each Other

Assumptions can have a grossly negative impact on your sex life. Learning to read signals and *checking them first* before reacting can save you years of heartache and dissatisfaction. Even for things you feel are positive, at some point you should ask to ensure you've interpreted his signals correctly.

I know a woman who believed her husband was very much into blondes, although she was a brunette. She would see him staring at platinum-blond women whenever they passed by them. One day she surprised him by having her hair bleached out to a pale platinum blond. When he saw her he was shocked. She was upset at his lack of positive response. A fight ensued with her asking him why he didn't like it when all she was trying to do was please him by bleaching it (she had never colored her hair ever before!) so she could look like all the other women he panted after. He was incredulous, explaining that he looked at those women because he was in awe of how unnatural and phony they looked! He adored how wholesome and beautiful his wife looked in comparison. She was crushed and immediately made an appointment to have her hair turned back to its original shade. Checking assumptions will improve every relationship in your life.

Be Honest with Your Man

Take responsibility for your own satisfaction—it is not up to him to read your mind! Face it: We don't build a house without blueprints. We don't bake a cake without a recipe. We don't start a business without a plan. Why then do we embark on a lifetime of lovemaking with very little idea of what we want, rarely knowing what our partners want, or how *we* can make us both happy?

Questionnaires you fill out separately and then share with each other may open up the doors to sexual communication. Keep the experience light, loving, and loaded with positive intentions. There are a few sample starters (delicious phrases) in chapter 20 to help you strengthen the foundation you've already begun to build. Following are some points to keep in mind when sharing thoughts on a potentially sensitive topic. These will help keep it a mutually safe and fun practice. These can be applied to any sensitive conversation with anyone.

- Location—keep it neutral, such as in a kitchen or while walking in a park. Discussions of your sex life should *not* occur in your bedroom.
- Timing—always check to make sure this is a good time. Stay away from "We need to talk," and instead ask if it's a good time or when might be a good time, since you have something you'd like to chat about.
- Stick to "I" statements. It's much better to say, "I feel this way when this happens" or "I want to have more romance and caressing," instead of "You make me feel awful when you . . ." or "You never touch me anymore." You are less likely to create defensiveness.
- Be clear of your intentions before you begin the conversation.

Marcia decided to bring some of her wishes and desires to Don in the hopes that she could become more satisfied:

I tried to keep things light and fun, even though I was crazy nervous. I made a brightly colored invitation and slipped it under his dessert dish after dinner one night. It said:

"I'd love to chat with you about some romantic ideas I've been having. Are you available for a cocktail in the den after the kids have gone to bed? I'm looking forward to sharing some kisses with you."

He didn't respond right away. We cleared away the dishes together and I tried to remember to stick with my intention to make things better for myself. Instead of getting upset or making demands of him, I kept cleaning up and thinking how great the evening would turn out. And it did turn out! If I had gotten defensive, I would have lost out on something special.

He opened a bottle of wine, took my hand, and we went to round the kids up. He took care of baths while I tidied up bedrooms and got pajamas ready. We shared reading duty and then went back downstairs. The wine had breathed long enough and was perfect. We got comfy in the den on the loveseat. I snuggled into him and we just enjoyed each others' company for a while.

Before I spoke, I checked in with how I was feeling, and really felt in my heart how much I loved him. I started out by telling him how I was feeling about him and us and how I wanted to make things spicier in the bedroom. I explained that I felt I was holding back some of my feelings and I wanted to start exploring more and asked if he would help me. I also shared that lace turns me on and that's why I had so many lace pillows in the bedroom. He sipped his wine, nodded some, and smiled. When I was finished, he gave me a huge hug and said he couldn't wait for us to get started. He said he respected me so much for sharing what was going on. He never really knew if I was fulfilled, but just assumed I was and was too uncomfortable to ask me about it. It was the start of a whole new period for us.

Encouraging Words

When it comes to sex talk in the bedroom, one of the simplest yet often overlooked ways to begin is to let him know when everything is just perfect. Especially in those precious few moments before your orgasm when you don't want him to move or deviate from the rhythm, tempo, pressure, or anything else—tell him! Make sure to let him know to continue just what he's doing when it's working.

If you want to get him to do more of something that you really enjoy, you can let him know by saying things like:

- ◐ "I love it when you go in deep."
- ◐ "It makes me crazy when you kiss my neck."
- ◐ "I go wild when you squeeze my butt."

This is a great way to educate him on your needs without asking him. He'll likely rise to the challenge.

My colleague Rebecca Rosenblat, relationship and sexuality therapist, TV and radio host, and author of *Talk Sexy to Me*, offers this wisdom on how we stand to benefit from learning the skill of sexy talk:

> *In being able to address our bodies without shame, we can eliminate the inhibitions forced upon us that go against our natural desire. If your mind can think it, your words can express it, making your sexuality as limitless as your imagination.*

●●● Kim's **QUICKIE TIP**

Teach him how to please you in bed. They say a picture is worth a thousand words. Imagine the words going through his mind as he watches you please yourself. This is sex education like he's never had!

Going Down a Different Path

If he is doing something you don't really enjoy and you don't want to stop the flow, you can do one (or all) of the following and he's sure to catch on:

- Say different things he does that you love (for example, if he's rubbing your tummy and it irritates you, say, "Ooh, I love it when you rub my back," and he's very likely to go straight for your back).
- Distract with a kiss so he stops doing what he's doing.
- Fine-tune your body position to one that works better.
- Gently move his mouth, hand, or whatever he is using to make it more comfortable or satisfying for you.

Alison had been enjoying her experimentation with Bill and was enjoying great progress seeing him stretch his comfort zone. The more she helped him out of his shell, the more she wanted to learn what he enjoyed:

I asked Bill if he was willing to play a game with me the next time we made love. He said, "Sure," and we ended up making love the following night. I started to purr as soon as he stroked my back. I've never purred before. I asked him if he could tell I was enjoying his hands all over my back, and he said, "Of course," because I was purring.

"Bill, would you be willing to moan and groan and yowl and purr to let me know how much you like what I'm doing to you?"

"Er, ah, okay, I guess."

Then I put my mouth over his beautiful penis and looked up at him. I swirled my tongue around and popped my mouth off with tight suction. He let out a small moan.

"That's what I'm looking for"

"Oh yeah, well, what sound do you make when I do this?"

He tossed me onto my back and nuzzled into my neck while squeezing both of my breasts. He knows I love my breasts squeezed. I started howling. We both giggled a bit, and then he put his whole body over mine and found my wetness. He pushed into me slowly and made some luscious sounds that I can't describe.

We continued on that night, making a lot of different noises. I really got off on listening to him. It seemed to bring out more of his animal side. I don't think we'll have too many more silent nights!

Sounds are very stimulating to the brain. Even the sound of panting or heavy breathing is arousing for many of us. The more you find your voice and let it out, the more he may reciprocate. Even if he doesn't, with you guiding him with your voice, at least he'll have a roadmap to what thrills you—even if it's an audio one!

Tone, tempo, and volume are also crucial to building a mood. A soft moan is different than a loud growl. A slow, deep breath is different than a sharp intake of breath or slower and deeper heavy breathing. A romantic whisper is different than a husky request for more or a deep-throated but loud demand to "get on your knees." Just like with sensations, build and vary the intensity of your sounds to create an erotic charge.

Have Fun with It

Make a game out of finding out what each others' signals are. Tell him what you believe he does to signal to you that he is feeling frisky. Ask him what he thinks your signals are. You may be surprised to find out you aren't exactly on target. Armed with new ammunition, you are more likely to prevent frustration! Look in chapter 20 for the "his and hers foreplay map" to do with each other. These are simple tools for improving how you interact in the bedroom. Surprises may be in store for both of you!

Practice Makes Perfect

Delivery is key. Become confident in your delivery and it will roll off your tongue like icing on a hot tummy. You don't want to be fumbling around while in the throes of passion.

You are unique. Take whatever step seems right for you. If you want some ideas of what to say to your lover, look in books, magazines, movies, or even ask him what you could say that would drive him crazy with lust! Or just go ahead and practice like Juanita did.

Being forty-five and looking ten years younger has always been a source of pride for Juanita. When she had her private practice, she could sway any jury in the courthouse. But it frustrated her that she felt so powerless in the bedroom. It wasn't that she felt weak staying home to be a mom to her two kids. It felt deeper than that.

> *How do you whisper something erotic to your lover that you have never said to another human being? First, I decided to practice in the mirror the way I used to when preparing for a trial. I don't want to be thinking about it while I'm having sex or it will just throw me off.*

I practiced making moaning noises so I could get used to the sound. It was tricky finding alone time, so I would do it in the car looking in my rearview mirror! I came up with some pretty sexy ways of asking him if he would hold me tighter. The night I first asked Carlos to take me from behind, I heard him suck in his breath and then I got an "Oh, baby!" that made us both pretty wild! All my practice built up my confidence. It was fantastic.

● ● ● Kim's **QUICKIE TIP**

Sexy letters, short notes, and subtle hints of what is to come can jump-start your sex talk.

SEXY CHALLENGE
Fantasy Presentation

You'll Need: Pen, paper, your creativity
Prep Time: Varies
Cost: $0
Raciness Factor: Bold
Benefit: Improves Communication

Invite your lover to write out his idea of the perfect sensual day of love and romance. Ask him to imagine giving you an exquisite day and evening to fulfill all of your sexual fantasies. Have him pretend money and time are no object. What would he do step by step? What are the details of any props to be used, foods to be eaten, the setting of the scene, clothing to be worn, the temperature, sounds, aromas, etc.? Have him write it out in as much detail as possible.

Then you do the same and write out what you feel would be a perfect sensual day for your lover. If you aren't comfortable writing it out on paper, you can e-mail or text each other. Perhaps you prefer to say it out loud as an audio message and record it or capture it on video. You can even sing it or draw it out if that works better. The key is to create a fantasy scenario for each other.

Arrange a time to present your fantasies to each other in creative and loving ways. Enjoy the freedom of make-believe and listen for all the glorious ways your man wants to please you.

chapter **9**

Position Yourself for Passion—No Yoga Master Needed

> Women need a reason to have sex.
> Men just need a place. —**Billy Crystal, actor**

Routine can get stale and boring. A favorite way to spice things up in your bedroom is to change the sex positions you use. You can prolong your lovemaking (and his orgasm) by switching to two, three, or even four different positions within a lovemaking session. Start with a favorite and excite your man by repositioning both of you for more advanced play.

This chapter offers exciting positions suitable for anyone. The fourteen positions on the following pages offer you the ultimate challenge of two weeks of great sex if you dare to try a new position each night!

To make things quicker and easier for you, here is a symbol guide to help you determine which positions to try first! Expand your repertoire, be flexible, and feel free to make up your own positions!

- **SS**—great for female self-stimulation
- **I**—perfect for when you feel a need for intimacy
- **C**—focuses on comfort for heavier people or those who have mobility concerns
- **DP**—useful for a shorter penis, since it allows deeper penetration
- **SH**—helpful for a longer penis, allowing shallower penetration
- **G**—wonderful for G-spot stimulation
- **1–5** is a scale for difficulty level (1 is the easiest, 3 is midrange, and 5 is the most challenging)
- **I–V** is a scale for fun factor (I is fun, III is tons of fun, and V is super-fantastic!)

Most women love positions where they are in control of the penetration. It can help them feel more confident so they relax and enjoy it more. Yoko added massage oil to one of these positions for a sizzling time:

I was feeling luxurious and very horny. I was squatting on Jim's tummy just playing around and I spied the massage oil behind the lamp on his nightstand. I don't remember the last time we even used it, but I reached over (he had to hold me so I didn't fall off the bed!) and grabbed it. I popped up the lid, held it upside down between my breasts, and looked into Jim's eyes as I squeezed the bottle. It was cooler than I thought it would be. Note to self: always warm oil in hands first!

Anyway, as it came out, I rubbed it all over my breasts

and my tummy and then wiped my oily hands on his chest and tummy. I put the bottle back on his table (closer this time) and then leaned forward, putting my breast in his mouth. He loves my breasts, so this was a big turn-on for him, especially with the almond oil all over. My tummy was on his chest and my pubic bone was on his belly button. I pulled my breast out of his mouth and we both moaned. I slowly slid myself down to meet his penis "head-on," so to speak. I started to rub my clitoris against his pubic bone, grinding a little, getting him more and more excited. I heard myself breathing heavily and almost growling imagining how great it would feel to finally have him inside me.

I lowered myself onto him, going only as far and as deep as I wanted to. I felt his strong arms around me and opened my eyes to see him staring intently at me with so much love. I came looking into his eyes. It was incredible.

Imagine how erotic it would be for your man if you were to keep his penis at your vaginal opening while you stimulated yourself to orgasm. Or if you were to plunge down at the moment of orgasm because you wanted him inside you when it happened. Be open to the possibilities for you both!

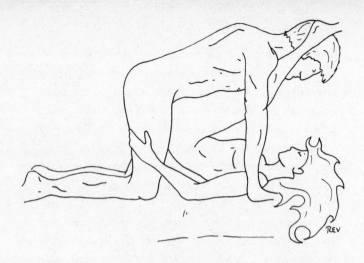

Modified Missionary
SS, I, DP, G, 1, III

Missionary position is the most common sexual position and was allegedly named by Christian missionaries who believed "man on top" was the only respectable way to have sex.

We call this one modified because her legs are up over his shoulders instead of down flat on either side of his. Have some extraordinary fun by adjusting the basic position of your man being on top of you by simply changing the angle of your body or either of your legs, which will change penetration depth. Try wrapping your legs around his back like a pretzel to help him go in deep and hard. Keep them straight down and tight so you are super-snug. If you're in good shape, hoist yourself up farther on your shoulders to give him an even more amazing, more intimate view.

Any position in which you face each other, enjoying eye contact, builds intimacy. Your hands are free for self-stimulation or for using a sex toy. What else can your hands do?

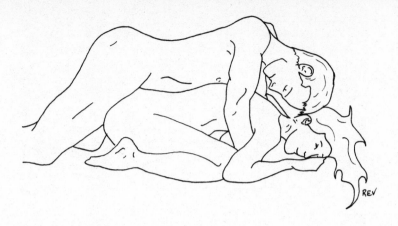

☼ Huddled Rear Entry
C, SH, G, 1, III

I suggest you try this with a man you trust, since you may feel a little less in control than with other positions. Start this position by being on your hands and knees and then slide your bottom back and down so your knees are resting comfortably against your chest. Then invite your man to gently lean over your back slipping himself inside you. For some women this position feels like a super-amazing hug! It's fabulous if your man is well endowed, since you can tilt your pelvis to control the depth of penetration. If he is heavy, modify this one so he is leaning back more on his knees with you adjusting yourself as required. If you can, reach back behind you to play with his testicles or perineum and he'll be moaning with delight in no time.

For variety, or if you just can't help yourself, you can push him up by rising up on your hands to grab the headboard or whatever may be in front of you, turning this into more of a typical doggy-style position. The secret is to do what moves you and, of course, whatever feels great!

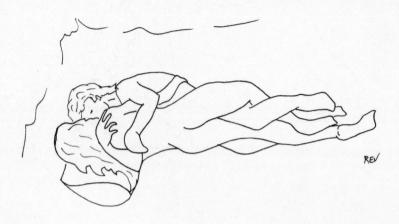

⬚ **Lovers Embrace**
SS, I, SH, G, 2, IV

I assigned this position only a 2 for difficulty since you might have a laugh or two until you find just the right combination of your legs up, over, or between that works best for the two of you. You can slip into this embrace quite naturally from the missionary position by both of you turning onto your side at the same time. Once there, you may find that sometimes it's easier if his legs are both between yours, or maybe if your bottom legs are both stretched out. Play with it! This embrace works for the G-spot as well, if you maneuver your bodies a bit to get just the right angle. Arthritis sufferers or folks who have mobility concerns find this one romantic and comfy. Again, you can control the depth of thrust, which is perfect if he's a bit on the larger side.

While you're in this position, take the opportunity to caress, squeeze, and touch your lover. This position is great for a Sunday morning before the kids wake up!

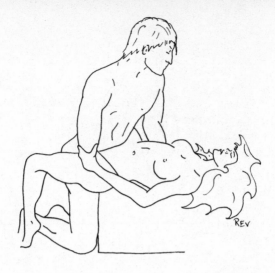

⬭ Furniture Lover
SS, I, C, DP, G, 1, V

Using furniture, such as a chair, bed, table, couch, desk, or bathroom sink, to prop yourself against makes for a feeling of very creative lovemaking. Try a set of stairs (use pillows to protect the back the person on the bottom!), leaning up against a wall, or bending over a comfy sofa arm to explode sex to a whole new level.

With Michelle's libido jump-started, she got back into lovemaking with an easy one:

> *I wanted to try a position where my extra weight wasn't between us or hanging down. This was great, because Dave really enjoys watching himself slide in and out of me, and I had some pillows propping up my head so I was totally relaxed and enjoyed watching Dave's excitement. Plus, my tummy lies out flatter. Next time I hope to get up the nerve to use my new vibrator at the same time!*

Risqué fun and comfort—what more could you want?

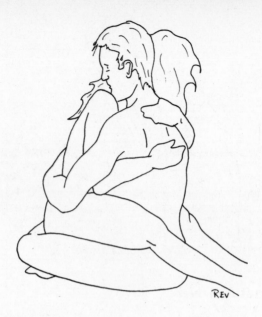

REV

⬡ Lover's Wrap
SS, I, DP, SH, G, 2, IV

What is more intimate than being opened up while face-to-face with your partner, with your legs wrapped around each other? The closeness is intense when in this position. Have your man sit up with his legs out in front of him. Then wrap your legs around either side of his torso and lower yourself onto his penis. This is one pose suitable for any penis size because you can achieve great depth by staying close in tight or sitting farther back for a more shallow option. Your hands are free to stroke or play with yourself, or you can invite your lover to play with you using his hands or a vibrator. Feel free to kiss long and deep while tugging on his hair, then nuzzle his neck and whisper sweet "somethings" in his ears. He'll be yours forever!

You may giggle or have to scooch together in a way that doesn't feel flattering, but the results will be worth it. From here, try lying back or pushing him back for even more fun.

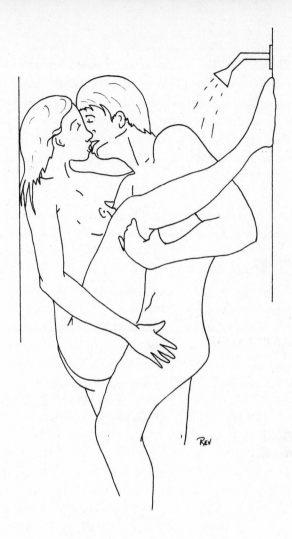

◌ Shower Steam
I, SH, 5, V

Yes, it's a rockin' good time, but can be a bit of a safety challenge. While facing each other in the shower, brace yourself against one wall. Have your guy lift up one of your legs as he slides himself into you. This steamy position works best in a shower *stall* so you can use the opposite wall (which will be much closer than in a typical shower) to keep your leg up, allowing your man use of both his hands to caress you. Alternatively, try resting your foot up on the edge of the tub for a variation that's still steamy. Juanita played with this position for one of her shower dates with Carlos:

> *I had been thinking all day of how I would take our bathroom date to a steamier level. The anticipation kept me wet even before I got into the shower. His back was to me as I washed it for him. When he turned around, I put my foot on the edge of the tub, leaned back against the wall, and asked him if he liked what he saw. I've never seen him get a hard-on so fast. I was already wet, so when he came to me, he slid in effortlessly. The power of his arms around me made me feel so loved. I arched my back and pushed toward him. As I moved my body he went with me, sometimes deeper, and sometimes he almost slipped out, but he kept his arms around me. I think I was actually close to an orgasm that time!*

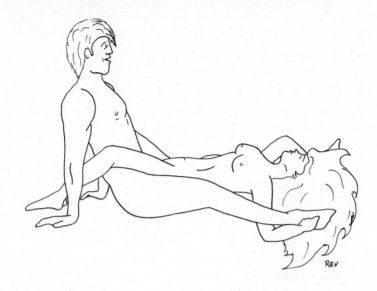

⦿ Backstroke
SS, DP, SH, 3, IV

Exotic. This position can make you feel like you're in a *Kama Sutra* movie. He sits up with his legs out in front of him. You straddle him and lower yourself onto him, wrapping your legs behind his back. This is the Lover's Wrap. Now have him grab your arms as you slowly lower yourself down so your back and head are resting on the bed (or floor or couch). If you reach back and grab his feet, you'll look super-exotic and he can pump in and out while you lie before him. Use your legs to squeeze him tight if you want to help him into you deeper. This becomes an intense visual experience for him, and you can enjoy using your legs as a sex workout!

A variation is for him to lie back while you stay upright or for you to both lie back together with only your genitals in contact. Experiment!

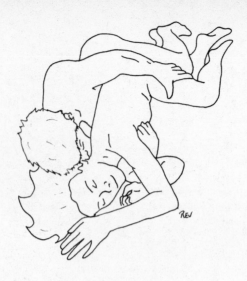

⠿ Spooning
SS, I, C, SH, G, 1, III

While not considered directly intimate because you aren't facing each other, you may find this position very romantic. This is another Sunday-morning favorite, lovely when you're tired or looking for some relaxing, gentle, slow lovemaking. You start out with both of you lying on the same side just snuggling together with him behind you. When you're ready, have your man slip his penis inside you and match his stroke or let him do the pumping action. It is a good position for G-spot access due to the rear entry, but if you stroke slowly, you won't have as much success as with other G-spot positions. Both of your hands are free; his for cupping your breasts and yours for self-pleasure. If you are pregnant, this is a delightful chance to have great sex while his penis doesn't go in as far (also great to try with a long penis). You can also relax and be more of the acceptor as he thrusts.

Add some variety to it by lifting your top leg back over his. He can even have his top leg bent up with his foot flat for extra thrusting power.

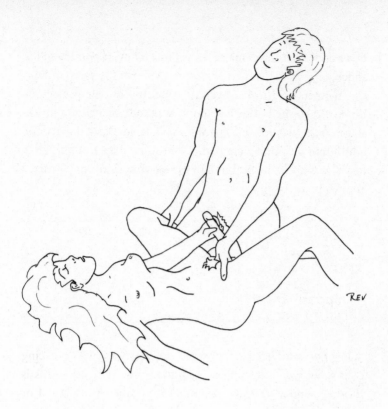

☼ Mutual Masturbation
SS, I, C, 3, V

This position is the safest sex you can have! While masturbation should be easy to do with and for each other, it may not come easily to you at first. That's why I've given it a 3 for difficulty. Also notice the top fun factor score!

You can pleasure yourself or each other. Most men are adept at pleasuring themselves, so watch and learn what he likes and how he likes it. Notice if he likes other areas stimulated, such as his nipples, testicles, or perineum. Some men will stimulate their anal opening while masturbating because it is loaded with nerve endings. Others may even venture a fingertip or toy in for added zing.

Women tend to be shyer about self-pleasure, especially in front of their men. This is a simple way to have a clean quickie and is great when birth control isn't available. Break down your inhibitions and build the path to intimacy. Use a blindfold at first if you find it helps, but aim for eye contact during orgasm. You won't regret it!

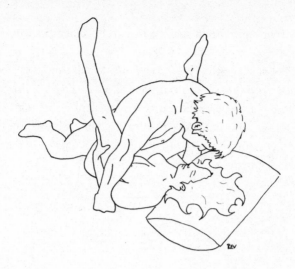

⬡ The Split
SS, I, C, DP, 1, II

The higher you put your legs, the deeper he can go, which is great if your lover is not well endowed. This is a variation of the missionary position. Here you lift your knees up and bring them back toward your head. Every few inches you move your legs can create different sensations for both of you. Wrapping your legs around him is also fun and helps you control the thrusting action. It may be awkward to use a vibrator on your clitoris if his torso is tight to you, so gently push him back and squeeze either your hand or a small toy in between the two of you and stimulate yourself to orgasm. He may enjoy the vibration as well as it may add another layer of pleasure.

This split is wonderful if either of you is heavy, since you have room to maneuver to increase pleasure for both of you.

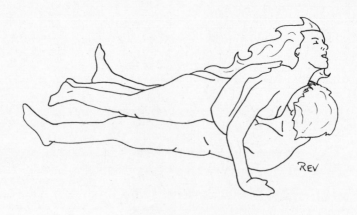

⋯ Floating
SS, I, DP, SH, 2, IV

This is a powerful position for a woman and not one often done. You'll likely surprise him with this one! Ask him to lay on his back with his legs open. Crawl seductively toward him, slide yourself on top, and lower yourself onto his hard erection. Lay your gorgeous body down the length of him ever so slowly and kiss him passionately. Rub or drag yourself up and down along his body to bring you the exact pleasure you seek. Grind against him so your clitoris gets just the attention it is looking for. Explore what happens when you close your legs tightly or use your legs to close his. What happens when one of you opens your legs again?

This position is a great bridge to or from sitting on top or even Reverse Cowgirl (see next chapter). You can float on waves of pleasure!

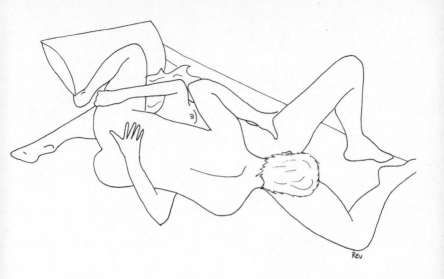

⚬ Side 69
C, 1, IV

Lying on your side using each other's thighs as a sensuous pillow is the start of this powerful entry into the category of 69. The traditional 69 position is done with one of you on your back and the other on top, with your heads to each others' toes. This can be not only awkward but also potentially uncomfortable for both partners. This version is far more cushy and relaxing. It also allows a more graceful way to pause to take a breath during all the activity. Most people find this position wonderful as foreplay but it is challenging to reach your climax while concentrating on the pleasure of your lover. On your side, you can more easily pause when you're close to orgasm while still caressing your lover with your hand or fingers.

Keep hydrated so your mouth stays moist, and enjoy each other!

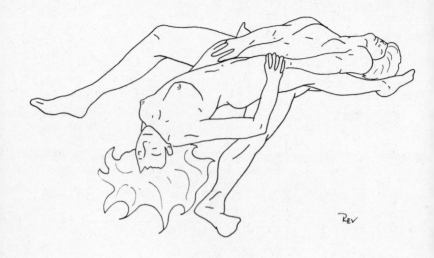

⬚ Sexy Scissors
SS, C, DP, 3, IV

At first glance, this may appear less intimate than some other positions. In fact, when you have your hands and bodies connected in this way, it is like you are one body moving to its own rhythm. Start out lying head to toe, then scissor your legs and direct his penis into your vagina. Clasping each others' hands gives you much easier leverage for going in and out, but will be a challenge if you want either of you to stimulate your clitoris. This position also works well if your partner doesn't get very hard erections. Either of you can use a free hand to squeeze the base of his penis to help maintain the erection.

You may have some giggles trying to find just the right angle to make this position work for you. Laughter is great medicine, even in the bedroom!

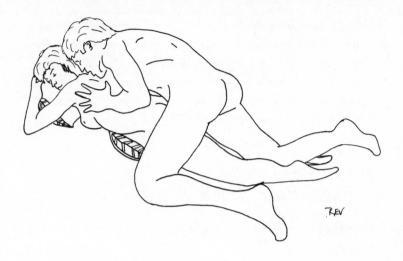

⦂ Sexy Sandwich
SS, I, C, SH, 1, V

This is potentially a very intimate experience even though you may not be facing each other. This position may be a huge turn-on if your man loves your butt. With you on your tummy, your man gently lies on your back with his penis either slipping into your vagina, your anus, or simply sliding snugly between your butt cheeks. Have a good, slippery lubricant available and feel free to push your buttocks up to reach him if you feel so inspired. If he isn't wearing a condom, be aware that if he ejaculates on your butt cheeks, some of the semen may drip down to your vaginal opening. He can crouch behind you or lay on top of you. The feeling of your lover's weight on you can make some women wild with desire. You may want to have a vibrator handy for yourself!

If you don't want him to penetrate you, this sexy position offers not only your butt cheeks but he can also slip his penis between your snug thighs instead for an "almost all the way" feeling. If he's more of a breast man, have him slide between your breasts with you lying on your back and him on his knees over you. You can help him along using your hands to hold your breasts for him. Alternatively, he can slip between your closed feet or even in your armpit. Explore!

SEXY CHALLENGE
Buzz, Buzz, Buzz

You'll Need: Vibrator and a sense of fun
Prep Time: None
Cost: $0
Raciness Factor: Bold
Benefit: Improves Sexual Skills

Try three positions you've never done before that permit easy use of a vibrator by either you or your partner. You can use it on your clitoris, his perineum, his penis, either of your nipples, or any other body part that is exposed and within reach. The novelty of the various positions will add some spice to your sex life and the toy will add some buzz!

chapter 10

G-Spot Secrets—The Map, Positions, and Techniques for Bountiful Booty

> If you really want something, you can figure out
> how to make it happen. —Cher, entertainer

Jen hadn't known about the Holy Grail of orgasms, but she found it on her first attempt:

> *When the G-spot was first explained to me, I was surprised and pretty doubtful. Lionel and I had never explored it because I didn't even know it existed. When I mentioned it to him, he said he'd heard of it over the years but figured it was a myth. He said he'd surprise me one evening and go on a hunting expedition for my G-spot. Well, he sure did!*
>
> *One night not too long ago he was giving me lots of love and attention and I was excited because I knew that we would make love that night. With his business undergoing some financial challenges, nights like this were be-*

*coming rarer. After the kids went to bed, we went upstairs
and he undressed me slowly while I stood in front of the
bed. He laid me back and kissed me all over, taking his
sweet time. It was heavenly.*

*Eventually he went down on me and slipped his magic
fingers inside, creating some amazing and wonderful twit-
tering feelings. I couldn't even tell where they were coming
from—it was so delicious. I started feeling something incredible coming up and outward from inside my core. Suddenly I felt a pressure like a contraction, only it felt really
good, and I just pushed down for some reason. Then this
wild explosion of juices came gushing out of me and all over
his face. I couldn't believe I'd had my first G-spot orgasm!*

Shall we start at the beginning? The G-spot as we know it was
named by Dr. Ernst Gräfenberg, who inadvertently discovered it
while he was helping women with incontinence (leaky bladders)
and helping them tone their pelvic floor muscles. He figured out
that some women derived sexual pleasure from stimulation of
the tissue of the urethral sponge. This "G-spot" is not in the
vagina, but is felt through the front vaginal wall, up and behind
the pubic bone.

There are two tricks to enjoyable G-spot play. One is to
urinate first, so you have an empty bladder. The pressure of a full
bladder may not be comfortable. The other is to make sure you
are aroused before you explore. The feeling of sexual pleasure
comes after the tissues and blood vessels of the area are swollen.
The ideal way for you to explore is to lie back on the bed. Have
your partner slip a lubricated finger inside you. Using the "come
hither" motion, have him apply pressure and crook his finger up
toward your belly button, scooping under your pubic bone.

The area may feel bumpy or ridged. It can be tiny like a pea
or bigger like a quarter. Usually it is felt at the top at the twelve-

o'clock position, but he may have to move his finger slightly to the right or the left. Let him know from your moans when he's found something new.

You can sometimes apply pressure to the outside of your tummy, over your bladder, to stimulate your G-spot, but it isn't quite as romantic or as easy to find that way.

Orgasms achieved through G-spot stimulation are often described as deeper and more full, "all over," and total, full-body-experience orgasms. A clitoral orgasm is generally more focused in the genital area and is often more intense. There are two nerve pathways in the pelvic floor that lead to the brain creating the sensation of orgasm, which may account for this distinction.

With all this talk of orgasms, it's important to note that the goal of G-spot play should *not* be orgasm. We all have this spot where swollen tissue surrounds the urethra. Not all women enjoy having it played with to the point of orgasm. Some ladies find it downright uncomfortable. The point, as with all sexual play, is to allow your body to let go and experience all the sensations associated with sexual activity and continue if it feels good and don't if it doesn't!

We'll cover the basics of the G-spot in this chapter as well as information on the best sex positions for G-spot fun, what toys work well for the G-spot, and the secrets of the male G-spot. If you want to explore further and expand your G-spot experiences, refer to my book *G-Spot PlayGuide: 7 Simple Steps to G-Spot Heaven!* available through www.kimswitnicki.com/greatsexforhardtimes.

G-Spot Orgasm

Women are often close to experiencing a G-spot orgasm when they make love, yet stop because they feel like they have to urinate. That usually means they're getting close! When you feel this pressure, bear down or push out and you may experience your first G-spot orgasm. Don't worry, you can't orgasm and urinate at the same time, because the urinary sphincter closes off the bladder when you climax.

Female ejaculation is a real occurrence and typically happens when the G-spot is stimulated. The liquid comes out of the urethral opening, not the vaginal opening, and is similar to male ejaculate without the sperm. It is thinner than vaginal fluid and often has a light, musky scent. There is anecdotal evidence of women expelling up to half a liter of fluid, but often it is only a few tablespoons. Relax. It is all quite natural!

●●● Kim's **QUICKIE TIP**

Keep towels handy when playing with the G-spot in case copious amounts of fluid gush out all over your sheets.

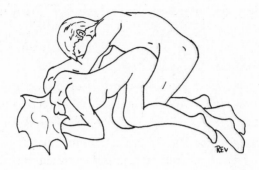

⬡ Doggy-style
SS, C, DP, G, 2, V

Rear entry is the best way for the penis to provide G-spot stimulation. Any position in which your partner approaches you from behind will work. With you on your hands and knees, your partner then kneels behind you and slips his penis in from there. You have the ability now to move your butt up or down to adjust the angle to suit your pleasure. In this position, the head of the penis is hitting the front wall of the vagina, where the G-spot can be felt. I have graded this a 2 because some women find it a challenge to be on their hands and knees and feel they are somehow being subservient or treated like a dog. In fact, it is so named because that's how dogs have sex. Check with your partner, but I'm sure he isn't thinking you're a dog at all!

You can modify this by propping your pelvis up on some pillows or cushions so you don't have to be on your hands and knees. All that's left for you to do is adjust the angle so it gives you maximum pleasure per push!

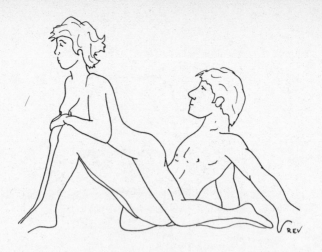

Reverse Cowgirl
SS, C, DP, SH, G, 1, IV

Not only is this sexy and will drive your man wild (since he probably loves to watch you), but it's totally comfortable and you can be more uninhibited since you can't see him watching you! With your man on his back exposing his lovely erection, stand over him with your feet on either side of his hips facing his feet. Gracefully squat down (this may be a challenge but he'll love it!) and guide his penis into you. Once you lower yourself on top of him, ask him to bring his knees up and adjust them for your comfort. He'll love that he can support you, and he'll surely enjoy the show.

You can modify this by going side-saddle or even leaning right back toward his head. The key to G-spot pleasure is different for each woman, since the man's erection is a factor. You control the penetration, so it is perfect no matter what size your lover's penis is. Move your pelvis around in whatever way feels most pleasurable. You can go up and down, rock back and forth, or simply sit right down and rotate your hips in a circular motion.

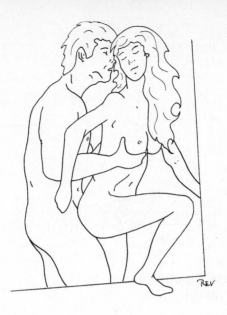

⠋ Leg Up
SS, C, DP, G, 1, III

The G-spot tissue does not have eight thousand nerve endings like the head of the clitoris. Because there are fewer nerve endings inside, you are more likely to have a response—hopefully a pleasurable one—to G-spot stimulation if you apply quicker and more aggressive thrusting of the penis rather than slow in-and-out action.

With your man penetrating you from behind while you both stand, raise a leg up onto a chair or a low table. In this position, both of you have your hands free to rub, caress, and stimulate any body parts that are available to you. Your one leg up allows for much deeper penetration. Play with how high your leg goes and notice how different it feels for you inside. Be careful, though, and make sure you have something handy to hang on to!

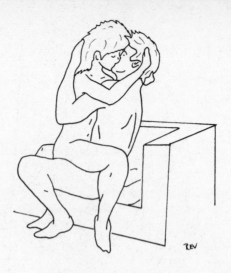

⦿ Lap Love
SS, I, DP, SH, G, 2, IV

This is one of the most intimate G-spot positions. Invite your man to sit on a couch or a chair while you then sit on his lap with your legs open to allow him to penetrate you. You can gaze into each others' eyes and snuggle together. You are also afforded the joy of your man stimulating your clitoris with his fingers while he is inside you. This is known as blended orgasm technique because he is stimulating both your G-spot and clitoris at the same time.

Being on top offers you the control you need to get the angle you want and also the correct depth of penetration. Either he can thrust in and out with you being still or you can use one leg on the couch or the floor to go with his rhythm or do the work yourself. Try another variation of this with both feet on the floor so you use the large muscles of both your legs—you'll tire less quickly—to propel you up and down. He'll love the fact that all he needs to do is sit there and enjoy!

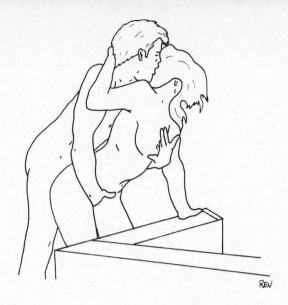

REV

☼ Urgency
SS, C, DP, G, 1, V

What makes this position special is that you can do it when you're in a hurry. Have your man penetrate you from behind while standing and you can lean slightly over a piece of furniture for support. You don't even need to remove all of your clothes! With the rear-entry positions, you get G-spot stimulation, and it adds a sense of "Take me, I'm yours" to the whole affair. Play with bending yourself over different couches or other furniture at different heights until you find the one that fits your comfort and joy criteria. Try grabbing his arm and wrapping it around your body. Take his hand and, with yours on top of his, fondle one or both of your breasts. You'll have him weak in the knees, so be sure to support yourself on the couch.

Use whatever furniture you're bent over as leverage to push yourself back into him and control the tempo. He'll love it when he feels you move this way beneath him!

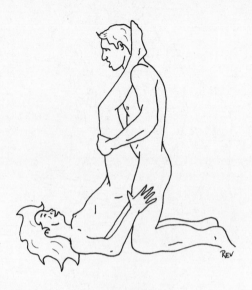

Modified Higher Missionary
SS, SH, G, 4, III

You will be at the mercy of your man and his strength with this much modified missionary position. While it can be a challenging arrangement to get into, it has erotic energy all throughout it. Position your man on his knees and have him pick you up while you face him. Wrap your legs around him and use a hand to guide his penis into you. Have him support you as you lower yourself back and down. You will look slim and trim as you stretch out before him.

If you try this with him standing, you can support yourself with your hands on the floor if that is easier for you. Let the blood rushing to your head be an enhancement to a strenuous but rewarding G-spot position!

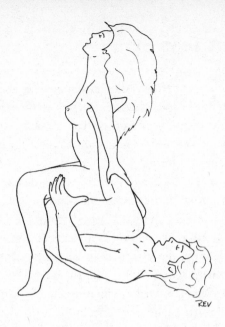

☼ Special Seating
SS, DP, SH, G, 3, III

Ideal for the active, brave, and adventurous woman who wants depth control and self-stimulation options, all while getting her G-spot stimulated. Have your man lie on his back and assume the "bicycle" position, lifting his butt and back off the floor with his weight on his shoulders, arms, and elbows. Slowly lower yourself onto his penis, resting your full weight on the backs of his thighs. If his erection is super-hard, this will be a challenge. If he can tuck his feet under your armpits, he can help support you. Rest against his feet for support and pump yourself up and down to your heart's delight.

Once you get comfortable getting into this position, you'll find it's fantastic, and that it's one you wish you had tried much sooner!

G-Spot Toys

Having great positions to try is an amazing way to explore your G-spot with your partner. Another way is to use a sex toy created specifically for G-spot pleasure. I highly recommend using the toy on your own first so you get comfortable with the sensations, but by all means if you want to dive in exploring with your partner—go for it!

What makes a great G-spot toy? A gentle curve is the key, so it can scoot up under your pubic bone to the G-spot area. It should also be rigid and hard instead of flexible and soft, since you need a firm touch and thrust to achieve the desired results. You must also like the look of it, since it will be involved in some pretty intimate activity with you! There are glass G-spot toys that don't vibrate, as well as vibrating models with curves and some regular-size shafts with large bulbs at the end to give you G-spot and clitoral joy. See chapter 12 for a sample.

His G-Spot

Men and women have analogous body parts. In other words, everything in the female anatomy has a match in the male. Men have a prostate gland, which is essentially the male G-spot. Even the tissue composition is similar to our urethral sponge. On a man, it is most easily accessed anally. As long as you use lubricant (men and women don't naturally lubricate anally) and don't force anything inside your man that he doesn't want, you may be able to bring about an orgasm for your man with prostate stimulation alone, without even touching his penis.

When beginning anal exploration, take baby steps first by gently running your fingers along his perineum (the oh-so-wonderfully-sensitive area between his testicles and anus) as part of manual or oral play. Try gently massaging the area and watch his face to see his reaction. Most men find this divinely pleasurable, since there are a lot of nerve endings here. When he appears comfortable with you playing in this area, consider using your tongue to stroll down the length of his penis, along his testicles, and under his scrotum. Then move along his perineum, licking and kissing. A shower first will help you both know he is fresh and clean! Push your tongue gently into his anal opening and feel him squirm with delight. You can also try using your finger or a small toy (order the Micro-Tingler from www .kimswitnicki.com/greatsexforhardtimes) and gently insert it into your man's anus as he nears orgasm. Not all men enjoy prostate play, but your man deserves to know if there is a whole new world you can both explore. If you meet any resistance, please don't force the issue. Trust, good hygiene, and baby steps are important for anal play, and a lot of couples find it incredibly worth the effort!

SEXY CHALLENGE
Gee Hits the Spot

You'll Need: You
Prep Time: None
Cost: $0
Raciness Factor: Regular
Benefit: Improves Sexual Skills

Keep you and your honey from playing with your clitoris in any way for three weeks. When masturbating or making love, engage in vaginal (G-spot) and other non-genital stimulation. Enhance your G-spot senses and see what happens.

chapter 11

Fabulous Fantasy—Imagination, Lingerie, and Role-Play Delights

Beauty is how you feel inside, and it reflects in your eyes.
It is not something physical. —**Sophia Loren, actress**

There are three areas of fantasy play that I will
outline here for you to experiment with. A large
component of great sex begins and even stays in the
mind. The first level then is about developing a sexually adventurous inner imagination that will, by itself, enhance your sex life. Let's also look at how
draping your body with negligee or other lingerie or
engaging in playacting with role play can turn an
already wonderful romantic life into a sizzling hot,
I-can't-wait-to-get-home type of love life.

Sharing Ideas

Sharing fantasies with each other is not only healthy
but also can lead to scorching sexual encounters,

even if you've been together for years. On the other hand, some fantasies are better left in the mind as kindling for lighting your own fire. As a rule of thumb, it is best not to share fantasies that involve having sex with your or your partner's family members, like siblings or cousins, or people you know, such as friends or next-door neighbors. Acting out these types of scenarios can be not only disappointing but also can cause permanent damage to cherished relationships.

Open yourself up to your lover with what turns you on, what would turn you on, and even what you think *might* turn you on. Being vulnerable and offering up your secrets can be a powerful, shared experience of trust. My friend and colleague Emaya Elfi Dillon is a sex educator and bodyworker and shares this about fantasies:

> When lovers choose to share their personal sexual fantasies, they reveal their deepest souls to each other. This increases sexual pleasure and can also enrich emotional intimacy and bonding.

There is nothing wrong with thinking of fantasies while you make love, if that helps you become aroused or reach orgasm. You don't want that to be your only source of pleasure, but the imagination is a powerful tool in the bedroom. Some couples enjoy whispering sexy scenes or situations they know will turn them on into each others' ears. Once you learn a fantasy or two from your man, try whispering bits and pieces of them into his ear while your hands roam all over his body and see what response you get.

We Respond to Visual Images

Visually stimulated minds create pictures that take us to new levels of erotic pleasure. Both men and women are aroused by visions of sexual romps and scenes of people indulging in sins of the flesh. However, men are usually affected most strongly by visual stimuli. It is often the man making love with his eyes open, watching his wife's face as he plunges in and out of her sweet body. She is blissfully unaware he is watching. Her eyes are closed as she basks in the glow of a sensual sun heating her up so she can float above the mountaintops.

Control Is in Your Mind

You don't necessarily have to share your fantasies before using them to add some spark to your satisfaction. You can imagine your lover is "taking" you and has you in his control without him actually knowing yet. Control is at the root of the most popular fantasy for women. The so-called rape fantasy is not about actual rape at all, but about giving up control and letting go of all inhibitions. Especially for women in positions of power or supervision at work, continual responsibility can be draining. If you are the primary parent, the one in charge of paying the bills, the one keeping the household organized, you too may have fantasies of simply being released from all duty and giving yourself over to someone else who is in charge. Juanita offers the following:

> When I learned that my fantasies of being overpowered
> were not only common, but they didn't mean I was weak
> or perverted, I was so relieved! I'm not sure yet how I'll
> bring it up with Carlos, but since he responded so well to

"Take me from behind" when I asked him to, I'm sure once I screw up enough courage, it will be fine.

Men may have similar fantasies of being overpowered, but the most common male fantasy is still a threesome with one man and two gals. They often imagine the joy of sleeping with twins, a mother–daughter team, or sisters, or you and your best friend. The reality is most likely best left in the mind as fuel for arousal and not actively pursued. Chapter 17 does offer you a safe way to test the waters of threesomes if it appeals to you.

Lingerie

The human body is a beautiful thing, and yet consensus has it that both male and female bodies are sexier with a little bit of clothing. Wear enough to leave a bit of room for the imagination. If you walk around nude, your honey will probably notice you as you walk by. If you walk around with a towel draped over your shoulder hiding most of the good bits, he is likely to follow you around! The tease can be more potent than the catch. You likely have a piece of beautiful lingerie way in the back of a drawer or in the closet. Take it out, dust it off, and surprise your man with a little fashion show. Try the Sexy Challenge at the end of this chapter for even more excitement.

Role-Play Fun

We loved to dress up when we were children, so why stop as an adult? Especially when the benefits in the bedroom are so fantastic. It may take a while for you to build up to costume play, but try baby steps first.

Consider adorning yourself in body jewelry or henna designs. Go for stick-on tattoos if you want to test the sexy factor without spending more than a dollar or two. Let your imagination soar with spectacular non-piercing body jewelry (follow the link on my Web site).

Jen enjoyed wearing a costume for Lionel, which helped her take on another persona:

I've always admired the famous stripper—or maybe she was called a burlesque queen—Gypsy Rose Lee. I borrowed one of my daughter's Mardi Gras play masks with fancy feathers, and I had a feather boa left over from a Hallow-een costume. One night when both kids had sleepovers, I put on the mask and some sexy music, wrapped the boa around me, and started dancing. Lionel was in his home office doing who knows what.

Even though I still had my regular pants and shirt on, I was feeling really sexy. I started to move in ways I imagined Gypsy would dance. It sort of took me over and my inhibitions seemed to take a vacation! After a while I noticed Lionel in the doorway to the living room. I'm sure he wondered what the loud music was all about. He was just watching me, mesmerized. The more I danced, the more Lionel watched and the more confident I became. Eventually he came over to me and we started dirty danc-ing together. We bumped and ground in ways that would put today's kids to shame. It was very fulfilling and one of those memories that gives me butterflies in my tummy whenever I think about it. Yes, we had some great sex that night!

Who Can You Become?

Costumes can be a great escape and can certainly help you feel sexy, but the real appeal comes through in *who* you are *being* when you are wearing them. As Jen realized, the costume accessories helped her get into the role of a Gypsy Rose Lee character, which in turn brought out the sexy dancer part of her. Jen's husband wasn't mesmerized by Jen because of the mask and boa but because he saw another side of her. What turned him on was seeing more of the sensual side of his woman come to the surface.

$ $ $ Kim's **CASH SAVER**

Convert an inexpensive set of wineglass charms into non-piercing nipple dangles by adjusting them snuggly around your nipples for an exotic look with no pain.

Great Deals

Halloween and Valentine's Day are great for spotting sexy costumes to wear for each other. Deals are to be found immediately after these two holidays, so that may be the best time to go shopping. You can try the costume rack at your local thrift store or even at the local dollar stores. True, it's mostly kids' stuff, but you may get lucky with something as simple as a wig and a sexy nurse's hat. Find some truly inspiring and sexy ideas at www .coquette.com and look up their masquerade line. Adult lingerie boutiques often carry the Coquette line. Simply devilish!

Kim's **QUICKIE TIP**

Your lover's closet also yields fancy costumes. Dress in each others' clothes and venture out for a hot night on the town. You may want to go to another city for this one.

In Preparation . . .

Often it is the building of suspense and anticipation that makes a planned sensual encounter oh-so-spectacular building desire to exquisite levels. Marcia spent weeks preparing for an elaborate night of love with her husband:

> I took a sexy picture of myself with our digital camera, printed it out here at home, put instructions on the back, and tucked it in the back pocket of Don's briefcase. In the photo I wore a blond wig from a prop shop in town and a pair of clunky old librarian glasses. I also wore the most boring business suit in my closet, but I left it unbuttoned and had nothing on under it so you could see half of my ample bosom. I wore lace panties, so I felt sexy. I had stockings held up with the garter from our wedding and I hiked my skirt up so you could see it. Thankfully I knew how to use the timer on my camera!
>
> After lunch that day I called him to say my folks were picking up the kids and were taking them out for dinner and would bring them home at nine. He thought that was sweet, and I could imagine he was figuring he could stay late at work then instead of coming home for dinner, since we like to eat as a family. Well, that soon changed when I put on my stern voice and said, "Don, I suggest you look in

Great Sex for Hard Times   **135** ❤

your briefcase in the back pocket. There is something there you need to see."

I was vibrating both from nerves while I waited for him to come back to the phone and from being turned on so much. He found the invitation with my picture. He came right back to the phone and said, "Marcia, what is this all about exactly?" with a tiny break in his voice. I told him in my stern voice again, "I suggest you turn it over, follow the instructions, and be here by four o'clock. Don't be late or I'll have to punish you." Click. I hung up after that and started sweating like mad. What had I done? Would he show up or was he right now thinking I'd gone off the deep end?

On the back of the photo I had written that I couldn't wait to have him inside me, that I was dripping wet with anticipation, and a few other juicy phrases that I thought would drive him wild. I also suggested he come home with something yummy to drink and an open mind and I would have candles, dinner, and a robe for him to wear. I asked him to think about the music that he wanted playing while I ravished his body and made love to him till he hurt.

He told me later how his hard-on kept getting in the way of his meetings and he couldn't keep his mind on anything but me! He left early and got home by 3:30—a record!

Costume Ideas

Think about what would be a turn-on for you and see what you have around the house to get you started. Lay things out in advance, even if only in your mind, so you are fully prepared. The anticipation alone is a sure way to get you purring. Costume suggestions:

- Nurse (white shirt, dress, a hat, and white stockings)
- Librarian (tied-back hair, clunky glasses, stuffy suit, unsexy shoes)
- Schoolgirl (kneesocks, pigtails, short skirt, blouse)
- Blond, brunette, or redhead wig (any color wig that is not your own)
- Cheerleader (pigtails, short tennis skirt, one of his jock shirts tied in a knot at your belly button, pom-poms)
- Maid (stockings, apron, feather duster)
- Cave girl (messy hair, old brown sheet cut up and wrapped like a toga, grunt your words)
- Cowgirl (cowboy hat, boots, cutoff jeans, bandanna, straw in your mouth)
- Businesswoman (briefcase with a sex toy and lube, classy suit with no blouse, bra, or panties, stockings and high heels)
- Superhero (old sheet tied around your neck like a cape with "Super Sexy" written on it in lipstick, stockings, your sexiest bra)

Next Step—Invite Him

Next you want to think of how to introduce the evening. Here are a variety of invitation options to get your creativity blossoming:

- E-mail or text it to him.
- Tuck a note in his coat pocket, pants pocket, or lunch bag.

- Call him before his day is over and send a fax.
- Have a file folder with a photo in it and drop it off at his office.
- Kidnap him from work while you wear an overcoat over your outfit.
- Tie a note around the neck of the family dog or cat.
- Fax it to his private line with no warning phone call.
- Send it in a pizza box.
- Put it in the middle of a bouquet of flowers.
- Mark a trail with the first note taped to his bathroom mirror.
- Put it in his morning coffee mug (before the coffee is in it).

Add a Picture

Adding a sexy photo of yourself to your invitation is pretty simple nowadays. Some photo options to use:

- Cell phone
- Digital camera
- Polaroid camera
- Photo booth at the mall (have a friend as a lookout if you're planning partial nudity)

Location Is Everything

If you can arrange a different location for your sexy scenario, do it to mix it up and keep him surprised. Here are some options for liaison locations:

If you don't have a camera with a timer, engage a close friend to take sexy pictures of you and you can return the favor for her so you each end up with sensual pictures of yourselves for your husbands (for a future date). Make sure you select someone you are comfortable with and who knows you well enough to allow your playful sex kitten to shine!

- Give him another address (switch with a friend).
- Go to an inexpensive motel to really make it a fantasy for him.
- Use your frequent flier miles or other reward plan points to get a hotel room.

Either way, taking charge in this scenario will leave him begging for more!

SEXY CHALLENGE
Sexy Photographer

You'll Need: Camera, modeling accessories
Prep Time: 15 to 60 minutes
Cost: $0–$20
Raciness Factor: Extreme
Benefit: Reduces Inhibitions

The aim of this challenge is not the photos themselves but the fun you both have in your roles. Let your inner shutterbug out to play (digital or Polaroid only please, for privacy). Take turns being both the model and photographer, capturing the passion of your lover on camera. Loud music can help get you in the mood. Accessorize your nude or partially nude body with a blindfold, silky scarves, a feather boa, a princess crown, opera gloves, stockings, a bathing suit, milk (to sip or pour over you), yummy fruit (to place strategically), stuffed animals, colored bed sheets, a blowing fan, books or magazines (to hold), pillows, exercise gear, and anything else you spy around you. Most of these items can be found in a dollar store or around your home.

Have fun coming up with ideas for each other using hobbies, sports you play, favorite pastimes, or fantasy images. Keep things light at first and, as you relax into it more, start to unleash your sensuality and offer more of your body (if you're the model) or ask to see more of your partner's body (if you're the photographer).

Location Options for a Pick-Up

Alternatively, spark some lust in your lover by having him pick you up at one of the following places. Dress the part and keep it simple and fun:

- In a bar or pub
- At a restaurant
- At a club or resort
- As a hitchhiker on the side of a road (beware of laws)

Role-Play Game

Invite voyeurism into your relationship by asking your lover to hide (if this works) in a closet and watch while you get out of a hot bath. Take your time drying off, applying lotion, lying down on your bed (or other convenient location), and pleasuring yourself to orgasm if it pleases you. Arrange ahead of time when you want him to come out of hiding. If it turns you on, switch roles!

> ♥ Some sexy scenarios take time, planning, and forethought. We easily spend time on our careers, health, what we eat, birthday parties, holidays, car maintenance, etc., so why balk at something as crucial to our well-being and our relationships as romance?

Secret Santa with a Twist

You'll Need: Paper and a writing utensil (can be a crayon, marker, paint—have fun!)
Prep Time: Depends on how creative you are. Enlist a friend to help if you want.
Cost: $0
Raciness Factor: Bold
Benefit: Improves Communication

Lingerie shopping is an erotic activity when done alone. Now you both have the chance. Go to a lingerie store by yourself (at a boutique, a mall, online, or through a catalog) and pick out something that you would secretly love to wear. Then create at least three clues you will give your lover that will point him in the direction of this fantasy piece of clothing. Don't use the size, color, or model number!

Try a short rhyme to have him figure out the color or use that color to write the clues. If he doesn't know your size, again try a rhyme or silly poem that repeats the number in it. Use a math problem if it suits you. If the size is simply a medium or large, have that word bolded in all of your clues. For the type, use another rhyme, poem, or clue that doesn't mention it directly. To get your creative juices flowing, here are some examples:

- **Panties.** "It covers my sweet spot. They can be for a granny or the beach."
- **Bra.** "Sporty cars wear them too. It covers the sweet-est 'pear.'"
- **Nightgown.** "Night on the town" (for rhyme). "The perfect 'slip into something comfortable.'"
- **Corset.** "It cinches, pinches, and makes me curvier."

- **Negligee.** "It'll make you have 'negligent' behavior."
- **Baby doll.** "Not for babies or their dolls."
- **Teddies.** "These little bears help children sleep better."
- **Bustiers.** "Makes my headlights stand right up."
- **Camisole.** "A sexy undershirt."

Invite him to visit the store alone with the clues to find your mystery item. Have him call you on your cell phone when he's done or secretly watch him to see when he thinks he has found it. You arrive and from there decide whether to purchase the item, try it on only (just for fun!), or simply enjoy admiring it together and celebrate him deciphering your clues. Go for a stroll hand in hand to get a hot chocolate and enjoy laughing about how much fun you had!

chapter **12**

Toys for Adults to Supersize Your Playtime

Sexiness wears thin after a while and beauty fades,
but to be married to a man who makes you laugh every day,
ah, now that's a real treat. —Joanne Woodward, actress

Laughter and intimacy go hand in hand. I spoke
to a couple recently who shared that, with two active
toddlers and two businesses, they weren't having
much sex, since there simply wasn't the time or energy. What really worked for them to maintain intimacy, though, was sharing little inside jokes, sharing
laughs about the funny things the children did or
said, and continuing to grab each others' behinds
when they passed in the hall. Not only is laughter a
great tool in the bedroom, it can lighten any stressful
situation and can build bonds that are unbreakable.

One surefire way to ensure you have fun in the
bedroom is to add toys. Playtime isn't just for kids,
and toys enhance a regular routine by adding a new
dimension. Mixing it up with variety in your sexual

antics is a key to longevity in your love life. If you have a new relationship (less than one year), you may not have a need for venturing into the toy arena just yet, unless you are already using toys and want something new to add to your collection. For those of you just starting out, give some thought to your reasons for wanting a toy.

Have a discussion with your lover or at least give yourself some quiet time to think about, or write about, what purpose you want your toy to serve. Decide whether it is for you alone, for both of you to use together, or a combination. Will it vibrate, and if so, for external clitoral stimulation, internal for vaginal penetration, or a combination? Do you have size or color preferences or allergies that could restrict the material it is made of, such as latex? You may simply want to find a game to play to boost your sexual communication or try a lovely massage oil for relaxing and getting in the mood.

Shop around for your toys to see what tickles your fancy. If you are at all unsure, seek an expert's assistance. A lot of shops and even online stores have staff ready and able to assist you. Some questions to answer before you make your first purchase:

- Is it for you alone or for you to use together?
- Do you want the option of penetration (this will affect size, texture, shape)?
- Does hard or soft material appeal to you?
- What material works best for you?
- Should it be waterproof?
- How quiet should it be?
- Would a realistic-looking penis or a smoother penis be better?
- Do you want it bumped, ridged, swirled, or smooth?
- How big would you like?

- Do you like soft or strong vibration, a range, or none at all?
- What colors work best?
- Do you want a game for fun, for romance, or to improve skills or confidence?
- Are there fragrances either of you like?

Most rubber, plastic, or glass toys do fine with hot water and soap to clean them. It is helpful to keep your toys in a toy bag or toy box so they are together, clean, and out of sight from prying little eyes, babysitters, in-laws, etc. If your toy is made of a porous material, or you are subject to frequent infections, or you are sharing your toy, an antibacterial spray will work best. Washing (or spraying) toys off after each use and storing them away for next time is all you need to do. You can find sprays at your local pharmacy or go to a sex toy shop or order them on-line. If you keep your toys in a plastic bag or plastic wrap, make sure they are completely dry after washing or else bacteria may form on the toy. A cloth bag or sealed box is best.

$ $ $ Kim's **CASH SAVER**

Sew a lovely piece of ribbon, string, or rope to the top of an old pillowcase and pop your toys inside. Tie it up and slip it over a hanger in your closet as a simple hiding spot.

Check out my Web site at www.kimswitnicki.com/great sexforhardtimes to start your toy exploring.

Note: Be aware of local laws regarding the purchase of sexual paraphernalia.

Vibrators, Dildos, and Dongs

Mention sex toys and people immediately assume you mean vibrators. You'll find vibrators with animal shapes and odd faces, in a rainbow of colors and textures, and with multiple speeds and functions. There is an array of smaller vibrators that you can put on your fingers or tongue, and even a whole vibrating glove. If you're willing to spend the money, remote control vibrators are sensational while dancing at a club or dining at a fancy restaurant. Take your time and figure out what you want—there is likely a perfect option for you!

The term "sex toy" is by no means restricted to vibrators alone. Yes, they are the popular choice, but there is a wide variety of items available to help you add new ingredients to an old recipe. I've sold sex toys since the eighties and they have come a long way with shapes, materials, and uses.

To be clear, dildos and dongs are penis-shaped toys *that don't vibrate*, and they're made from materials such as rubber jelly, latex rubber, vinyl, PVC, glass, plastic, and silicone. These are primarily designed for penetration into the vagina or anus. You can also find them made out of wood, metal, stone, leather, jade, and other materials, but these are usually art pieces or are relics from ages past. Yes, sex toys have been around for centuries!

Vibrators *vibrate* and are primarily designed for external clitoral stimulation or internal G-spot stimulation, though they are often used on other areas of the body as well. They are usually made of the same materials as dongs. There aren't too many arty vibrators, though. At the historical adult ladies boutique Eve's Garden in New York City, there has been a lovely pink collector's vibrator that is a piece of designer art—brass stand and pink case included! The battery-powered models (which used to only be available to medical professionals) have been around since the late 1800s. These tools can save time, tongue muscles, and can prevent tendonitis of the forearm!

When using a vibrator, you can:

- keep it still and steady in one delicious place on or near your clitoris
- employ a press-down-and-let-go action
- rub it around your pleasure zone
- move it back and forth
- hold it on your man's frenulum (see chapter 3)
- stimulate his testicles
- use it to massage other areas to relax
- use it in any other way that brings you or your lover pleasure!

The most common type of vibrator is typically used for clitoral stimulation. I prefer multispeed so you can control the intensity of the vibration depending on how close to orgasm you are or what mood you're in. Some women like to have the option of penetration with their vibrator, so it is nice to have your toy shaped like a penis. A lot of men enjoy watching their women

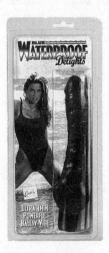
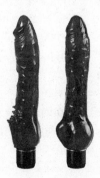

be penetrated too. The softer the material, the more it will absorb the vibrations, so a firmer toy is better if you need or want stronger stimulation. The one on the previous page has some extra bumps and ridges at its base to give you a bit more stimulation of the vaginal lips and clitoral area when it is fully inserted!

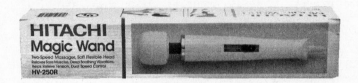

The strongest vibrator currently on the market is the larger, less phallic-looking vibrator, the Hitachi Magic Wand. For over thirty years it has been recognized as a premium sex toy and is the most common toy used by sex therapists to help women who are pre-orgasmic. The original is a plug-in model, though you may find versions of it that are rechargeable. It can't be used for penetration (though there are attachments for G-spot play) but the two-and-a-half-inch flexible head will deliver stronger sensations than any other toy. If you need strong sensation or have trouble achieving orgasm, this may be your answer. It can be used on sore back muscles too!

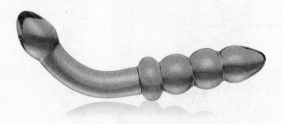

The sleek look of a glass dildo induces people to purchase one for aesthetic value alone. Often they have swirls of color in them and don't look like sex toys at first glance. I have a client who insists hers is a work of art and she proudly displays it. Glass dildos (and yes, you can get glass vibrators too) can be warmed or cooled using hot or cold water, which provides interesting sensations when rubbed along your vulva or inserted inside you. Don't knock it till you've tried it. The one on page 150 is curved for G-spot play.

Glass is also the most hygienic material used for toys (such as the one shown here) because it is nonporous, so it doesn't absorb bacteria. It's also a lovely inert material, useful if you have latex sensitivity or if you're prone to infections. It provides easy cleanup too because it's dishwasher safe. If you have kids, you may want to put this load away yourself! Because they aren't porous, lubricant isn't absorbed into them, so they stay slippery when lube is applied. Made from Pyrex, they shouldn't break or chip during normal use and usually come with a fabulous lifetime warranty.

● ● ● Kim's **QUICKIE TIP**

Place some ice chips in a Ziploc bag and keep it in the freezer to take out when you want to use your glass toys.

One of my favorite toys is this narrow little slimmed-down bullet called the Micro-Tingler (as shown on page 152). It is three inches of silent power that enhances masturbation, oral sex, intercourse, and anal play. Due to its small size, it's a great way to introduce toys into your relationship. If you have a sexy little toy like this inserted into your vagina while making love, your husband is making love to a vibrating vagina, which can be a unique and erotic experience. Play it along your cheek while performing oral sex. Its small size makes it perfect for exploring anal pleasures. You can listen to an audio description of how to use this toy on my Web site (www.kimswitnicki .com/greatsexforhardtimes).

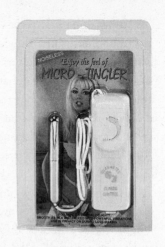

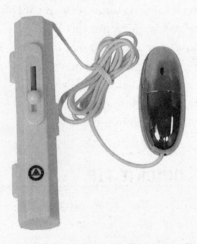

These magic bullets (above) can also be inserted inside your vagina—two at once for a more "full" feeling!—but they may be a bit too big for use clitorally while you are having intercourse. It can be done, but be watchful of pubic bone bruises. Magic bullets work best for self-stimulation, and a lot of women swear by their silver bullets and don't go away on holidays without them!

When you take a vibrator with many different functions, such as different speeds, pulsing, and escalating modes, and add a shaft with beads that rotate and then add a clitoral stimulator with many different functions, the result is a whole new world of fun! Made famous by *Sex and the City* (remember the episode with the rabbit vibrator?), these deluxe, multifunction vibrators allow for amazing opportunities. It's not recommended for a first-time toy purchase, but if you want to start at the top, be prepared for an intense adventure. Blended orgasms, anyone?

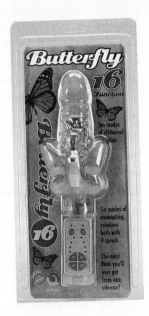

● ● ● Kim's **QUICKIE TIP**

Always keep spare batteries in your bedside table, purse, and suitcase, because you don't want the buzz to stop at that special moment!

Lubricate the Wheels

To keep both your and your man's engines humming, I believe the most necessary sexy accessory is a water-soluble, flavored lubricant. If you've never made any accessory additions to the bedroom, I suggest a bottle of lubricant in your (or his) favorite flavor. Multipurpose accessories (you can use flavored lube for oral sex too) really bump up the booty factor in your bedroom. Michelle is now a fan since she bought some in Dave's favorite flavor: JuicyFruit (available on my Web site). She loves the slippery feeling she gets with it for intercourse, and Dave has started performing oral sex on her again!

Balls, Rings, and Pumps

When we are younger, our bodies tend to do more of what we expect of them. As we age, our pelvic floor muscles become weaker, and both men and women can develop health issues that impact our ability to function sexually at optimal levels. Stress can play a role as well, creating health issues for us in the bedroom. The sex toy industry has provided us with some solutions for our various frustrating functions so we can continue having great fun while enjoying great sex.

Ben Wa balls, the gold-plated metal balls pictured here, are designed to be inserted vaginally for muscle tightening (to perfect your Kegel technique), which will improve the strength of your orgasms and help prevent incontinence. You work up to keeping them in for about fifteen minutes a day to tone your pelvic floor. For a nontherapeutic use, make love with them inserted, using gravity to your advantage, and move from one sex position to another. They will move slightly within your vagina and may help stimulate nerve endings deeper inside you to bring you previously unknown gratification.

A word of caution: inform your partner if you have them inserted, in case he decides to perform oral sex on you; you don't want to have to perform the Heimlich maneuver or have to rush for emergency dental surgery when you're wearing your sexiest negligee!

You can also find vaginal pumps, which are like suction pumps designed to suck on the vulva area—quite arousing for some women, and some men enjoy the look of a plumped-up pleasure center.

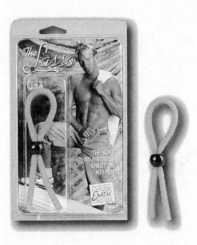

Your basic erection ring (also known as a cock ring) is for men who can achieve an erection but have trouble maintaining it. Slide the ring over the penis all the way to the base using some lubricant or saliva. Gently tighten it, preventing blood from flowing back into the body so the erection will stay hard. Don't keep the ring on your man for longer than thirty minutes at a time. There are also rings that have small vibrators built in.

The ring will not delay orgasm for him, but may help him keep his erection, may also bring on his orgasm earlier, and if he wears it with you, the extra stimulation can help you be more orgasmic, which should keep both of you happier!

When men have trouble achieving an erection, they can try using a penis pump. These pumps use a vacuum pumping action to bring blood into the penis, creating an erection. This is a temporary fix, yet can be great help if you don't mind using the pump each time before you make love. Many men want larger penises and believe these pumps will do that. It is possible, but takes a lot of effort over a long period of time. Most women are more than thrilled with the current size of their man's penis. It really is what you do with it that brings women joy.

Potions

A myriad of gels, lotions, and potions has been created to enhance your lovemaking experience.

- If you don't enjoy your man's taste while you're performing oral sex on him, you can buy Good Head or other tasty gel to sweeten up the fun.
- For women who need an extra boost to get in the mood, there are clitoral stimulation gels for topical application to the clitoral area, creating blood flow, swelling, and heat sensations. It's hard to think about soccer practice and grocery lists when you have a warm and tingly sensation, giving you shivers and quivers between your legs.

- Edible body paints are a hoot for creative types to design a work of body art. The best part is licking it all off afterward.
- Massage oils and massage bars (some are even edible) can add romance and intimacy back into a tired relationship. Touching not only is therapeutic, it can remind you both of your love, even if you are tired, stressed, or not feeling well. It doesn't have to lead to sex, so incorporate regular massage into your relationship, even if only for five or ten minutes.
- I don't recommend gels that claim to make you tighter or that will enhance your G-spot sensation. Always carefully read ingredients to ensure that you know everything you are putting in your body. You're much better off learning how to do proper pelvic floor exercises for tightening and experiment with your G-spot, which is why I created my DVD program for bladder freedom and my *G-Spot PlayGuide*.

$ $ $ Kim's **CASH SAVER**

Use chocolate syrup, jam, icing sugar, or cake sprinkles to decorate your lover instead of buying body paint from a love shop. Keep the sugar away from the vagina, but the rest of you is available for decorating.

Michelle chose Kama Sutra body care products to get reconnected with her sensuality:

Because it had been so long since I really felt like a woman, I started doing small things to get back into my sensual groove. I started taking luxurious-feeling bubble baths with scented oils and bath salts. I had some old Honey Dust, silky, honey-tasting powder from Kama Sutra, underneath my bathroom sink of all places and it was still good! I started dusting myself with it after my baths, and the feather applicator rolling around my body helped me feel romantic.

My friends and I are constantly giving to our husbands, our kids, our families, and each other, but we don't take time for ourselves or even treat ourselves. Yes, a mint shower gel may seem like a luxury to some, but for me, I'm starting to get back the womanhood I thought was gone forever. I'm totally worth it!

Swings and Games

There are lots of wildly fun games you can play to connect, to find out more about each others' turn-ons, to use as foreplay, and simply to have fun. There are card games and dice games and complete kits of fun complete with accessories such as massage oils, feather ticklers, instruction cards, blindfolds, and more.

Here are a few options:

- Sexy dice, where every roll is a winner, matching a body part with an action
- Card games, such as Fore-Playing Cards or strip poker
- Handcuffs, with or without fur, for bondage play—don't lose the key!
- Edible underwear (These can be an entertaining way to drive your sweetie crazy as he gets turned on while you nibble away. Beware of panties with licorice

strings and material made from candy sheets. They are very sticky when wet and can get stuck in pubic hair. Not sexy! I suggest the string bikinis made of candy rings, as they are much more user-friendly.)

- Velcro bondage kits (These can be an exciting way to ease into more risqué play. The ankle and wrist restraints for attaching to bed posts or chairs are made with Velcro so you can "escape" if you really want to. For more on risqué play, see chapter 19.)

- Feathers (Chapter 20 has a link to your free copy of my Lioness Deluxe Sexy Feather Game for hours of erogenous zone discovery.)

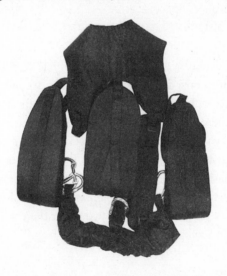

The posh sex swing above is something you acquire when you already have one of everything else! It allows you to access more extreme sex positions and is also a treat if you are arthritic or have muscle restrictions. There are a few different love swings on the market, so do your shopping. All you need is a ceiling hook, a load-bearing beam, and an appetite for trying out lusty positions. This is an investment in sexual furniture—and what a wonderful workout!

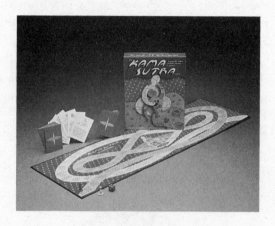

The Kama Sutra game (shown above) has been a favorite of my clients for years. Sexual board games for two are a great way to initiate love play. They also may help open lines of communication. The one above is designed to help you connect on a deeper level with your lover and is especially good for reconnecting lovers in long-term relationships. Board games are an easy way to initiate foreplay and to find out more about what makes the other's heart go *thump*, *thump*, *thump* with desire. Lay out a big, soft blanket on top of your bed, light the candles at your bedside, dim the lights, and let the games begin!

Toys for Two

While some toys can be used by yourself alone or with a partner, there are some designed exclusively for two people. For example, there is a whole line of strap-on toys made originally for gay women or men to penetrate their partners (using a dong or vibrator in a harness strapped to your waist), but more and more heterosexual couples are expanding their sexual experiences to include the joys of strap-on play as well.

Vibrating cock rings may be used by men for masturbation, but are also designed to be used during intercourse with the woman on top so she can control the "where" and "how much" of the vibration. Double-ended dildos (a long dildo with a head on either end) are often used by gay women, but can also be enjoyed by one woman inserting it into both her vagina and anus for a very full feeling, or by an adventurous couple wanting anal penetration for him and either vaginal or anal penetration for her. The longer the toy the better for achieving maximum flexibility.

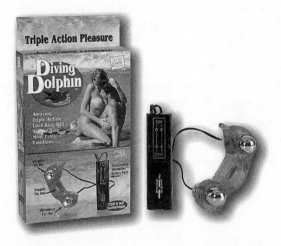

A favorite with couples since the seventies, the Diving Dolphin is worn like a cock ring and has two vibrating bullets. It will have you giggling while you try to find the best way to situate yourselves. "Woman on top" is the most common position to use this toy, since you have better control of the amount of clitoral stimulation from the dolphin's nose. The other bullet offers stimulation for either your man's testicles or your anus. The bullets can be removed and used for either clitoral or vaginal stimulation while making love. This is a surefire way to add some excitement to your routine. Let him hold the controller—he'll love watching you squirm!

$ $ $ Kim's CASH SAVER

Enter code GSHT when you order any of the games on my Web site and receive a 20 percent discount—another gift for you!

And So Much More

A wide range of anal toys awaits those adventurous enough to explore (see chapter 19 for more on anal play) such as special anal vibrators, anal beads (to be pulled out during orgasm), and butt plugs, which range from small to large and are flared at the base for safety so they don't get "stuck" after being inserted. You can also find double-pronged vibrators for the vagina and anus, with the anal prong being smaller.

Men can use penis sleeves for masturbating (often called "pocket pals"), penis extensions for length and girth, and French ticklers. A tickler consists of a rubber penis sleeve with wiggly bits attached at the end purported to stimulate a woman inside, but our nerve endings really aren't that sensitive deeper in the vagina, so the ticklers mainly just look cute.

To dress up your body, try non-piercing body jewelry for nipples, your clitoris, and even your vaginal lips. Cock circlets are stunning jewelry on a penis for decadent decoration. Vibrating and non-vibrating clamps are designed for all sorts of body parts too. Whew! As you can see, this chapter is only a taste of the escapades that await the brave and curious.

SEXY CHALLENGE
Toys for Two

You'll Need: One of your sex toys
Prep Time: None
Cost: $0
Raciness Factor: Regular
Benefit: Improves Sexual Skills

Use one of your sex toys in a new way. This can be you on your own, using a different speed on your vibrator or starting your self-play on areas of your body you don't typically stimulate. If you have a vibrator, bring it into your couples play and use it on your man on his back, butt, or perineum and see what develops. Then ask him to use it on you in a way he's never tried before.

SEXY CHALLENGE
Sexy Stash

You'll Need: Sexy stash items, velvet or other type of sexy bag
Prep Time: 15+ minutes
Cost: $0–$20
Raciness Factor: Regular
Benefit: Increases Inner Sensuality

You may already have a cornucopia of sexy goodies around your home to stash away in a few secret sexy places. Remember the velvet toy bag idea from chapter 5? You or your man may initiate lovemaking more often when you both know the secret location of your hidden bag of treasures. Marcia was thrilled when she created hers:

> *With three kids roaring around the house, it's nice to know I have a few tricks up my sleeve that they don't know about. I didn't realize how many sexual items I already had. I keep sex more in my mind now too, because I always see new, fun, spicy things to put in one of my goody bags!*

Create a sexy toy bag to stash wherever seems best to you. Try some of these ideas to get you started: a feather duster (for tickling), stockings, a scarf (as a blindfold), dish soap (for bubble baths), a hairbrush (for exotic skin sensations), or flavored lip gloss.

Add items that provide a visual treat, such as costume pieces (a feather mask, a nurse cap, glasses, pigtail ribbons, a cop hat, a bow tie). Remember the other sensual senses such as touch (something soft to the touch or lotion), smell (potpourri), taste (candy cinnamon hearts), and hearing (sexy CDs or iPod) when you are rounding up your treasure trove. Create a full-on sensory experience!

Don't forget to let him know where the stash is as well—or send him on a scavenger hunt to find it. Reward him well when he does.

chapter 13

Mouth Magic—Oral Sex Tips to Make Each Other Ache with Anticipation

Each kiss a heart-quake. —**Lord Byron, author, *Don Juan***

Oral pleasures are opportunities for one of the most sensual and intimate affairs you can have with someone you love. Formally called fellatio if performed on a man and cunnilingus when performed on a woman, if you can become master of either, you will be revered. Some people are intimidated by the thought of performing orally, and yet others consider it a mere extension of kissing. So whichever you are, consider yourself normal. This chapter will arm you with tricks, techniques, and many erotic ways to use your mouth to make your mate melt. Once you become comfortable and confident with pleasing your partner in this way, you will have him eating out of your hand—so to speak! Hopefully, you will have this delightful oral expression of love reciprocated. It is powerfully intimate to kiss your sweetheart in this way. Before we get into the specifics, here is how Juanita stepped up to set the scene for a night Carlos will never forget:

Carlos loves it when I perform oral sex, but I have mixed emotions about it. I resolved to set up an evening that would really work for me so I could let down my guard. Everyone thinks I'm so confident about everything and they have no idea that I have these hang-ups about sex. Oral sex doesn't usually do much for me, which is frustrating for both of us. I've opened up a lot, learning how to use my voice and make more noises, which has been fun, but I still have a way to go.

Setting the mood with dim lights, cherry-scented candles that he loves, and some of his favorite music on the stereo helped put me in the mood for romance. He was out at a dinner meeting, so I wanted him to relax when he came in the door.

When he arrived, I greeted him wearing some lingerie he had bought for me years ago, and I don't think I'd ever worn it. I had to rummage around the back of a few drawers before I found it! I kissed him passionately and told him the kids were out and wouldn't be home for a few more hours. I felt him growing hard as I kissed him slowly and then with more urgency. I undid his tie, swirled it off him, and started undoing his shirt while his hands swarmed all over me. I've kept myself in great shape and know he appreciates my body.

I'd just learned about the "M-zone"—the area going up both of his front thighs almost to his belly button and then down to a point at his penis—from an oral sex class that I took, and decided to test it out. I nuzzled his hard-

ness through his pants with my mouth and then switched over to his right thigh. I got frisky, biting him softly through his wool dress pants, all the way up his thigh as my hand squeezed the other leg. My mouth and hand met at his belly button and I flicked my tongue around it. He quickly removed his shirt and held my head to move it up toward his face, but I resisted. Instead, I went lower again, down to his belt and the edge of his pants.

His breathing was getting hoarse as I undid the belt with my hands and the single button slipped quickly through its hole as my teeth pulled at the fabric. Then the zipper came down achingly slowly, since it was pushed tight by the rather large bulge in his slacks. His anticipation of my mouth being on him was making him crazy and that started to turn me on too. I was in charge here.

I paused. I slowly made my way back up his stomach with my mouth giving small kisses and tiny love bites and occasionally flicking my tongue. Meanwhile my hands were rubbing and caressing any parts of his body I could reach at that moment. When I got to his right nipple, I lazily circled my tongue all the way around it once, twice, three times. This was my show. I could see that prolonging the main event had him ready to burst. I tiptoed my tongue to his nipple and held it between my front teeth. He sucked in his breath. I gently squeezed my teeth together and he moaned so loudly I was startled. His mouth was close to my ear, so it was loud! I lifted my left leg and wrapped it behind his and then suckled his nipple while my left hand reached down to his crotch. I thought his legs were going to buckle. He hoarsely said, "Juanita, you're making me crazy here!"

I was so turned on at this point that I dropped to my

knees and yanked his pants down around his ankles. He was so swollen and hard. It only took a few minutes and it was all over for him. It was the shortest blowjob I'd ever given, if you only count the part where his penis was in my mouth, but I know he'll never forget it!

It's amazing how some knowledge and a bit of practice leads to buckets of confidence!

Seize the chance to get your whole body into the oral sex event. Juanita used her legs and hands and not just her mouth. She also set the scene with elements she knew her man enjoyed. Adding in massage oil and rubbing parts of your body on your lover will do nothing but heat things up. Add in some teasing and playing with other erogenous zones like nipples, buttocks, the scrotum, thighs, arms, or feet and you have the makings of some very memorable moments.

Ideally, when it comes to oral sex, you aren't simply putting your mouth or tongue on your lover's genitals, you are *making love* to the penis (or the vulva). The goal isn't just to have him in your mouth but to drive him wild by licking, nibbling, sucking, caressing, fondling, playing with, and generally stroking *all* his pleasure zones. I'll get to some yummy specifics on how to do this in a moment. For now, the important thing to realize is that the more you enjoy yourself, the better the experience will be for him! It will drive him to the limits of sexual desire if he can tell you are into what you are doing. If he thinks you don't like what you're doing or are really embarrassed or uncomfortable, it won't be much of a turn-on. However, if you feel hot and sexy and are treating his penis like a decadent treat you've been craving, you can't go wrong and you can only improve the more you do it!

Guidelines

First, a few general rules . . .

Squeaky clean is the rule for any oral play. Our bodies' natural musk and other aromas can be a turn-on for some, but start with a sparkling fresh foundation, because arousal will enhance your natural scents. Hygiene is also important to prevent bacterial infections. We usually feel much more comfortable when we are clean. Not many men or women are relaxed having someone start kissing them all over when they don't feel clean.

Note: Ladies, if we aren't clean, there is a greater chance of picking up a urinary tract infection, since the urethral opening and rectum are close together and an active tongue or finger can move bacteria into the urethral opening unintentionally.

The absolute most important factor in oral sex is communication. Am I repeating myself? Communication is an invaluable tool, so learn to listen to your lover's voice, moans, breathing, and even heartbeat if you're close enough to his chest. Learn to "hear" how close he is to orgasm so you can either delay or prolong it, depending on what your aim is. You can use your ear to tell if you should vary the pace or the stroke. If he has gotten quiet, he may not be enjoying himself as much. It's always best to check in with him while you're developing the skills of reading his body's signals. A simple "Should I go faster?" or "How would you like me to continue?" can give you helpful information.

Also watch to see the expressions on his face or if he is squirming in discomfort or absolute bliss. Taking in all of the visual, auditory, and sensory signals—e.g., is he getting hard like he does just before orgasm?—can take some practice. Hopefully you'll have a lifetime together to hone your techniques!

I Have His Penis—Now What Do I Do with It?

If you follow the guidelines in this chapter, are gentle with your man, and communicate, you can't go wrong. Most men love oral sex. Some even enjoy it more than intercourse because they get to lay back (or kneel or stand) and have you do all the work!

- Make sure you are in a comfortable position, since you don't want to spoil the mood with a leg cramp or develop a kink in your neck. If he is on his back, find a comfy spot down between his legs. If he is on a couch, standing, or sitting on the edge of the bed, you can be on your knees before him so he can see all the action.

- Keep him lubricated with your own saliva or use a nice flavored lube. Slippery is almost always better than dry.

- If you are using oral sex as foreplay and your man is soft—can you say midnight or early-dawn surprise?—this is the time when you are most likely to fit him all into your mouth at once. Gently place your mouth over his penis, wrapping your lips around the base. Apply gentle pressure with your lips (remember, no teeth—ever!) and slowly bring your mouth up to the top. Your thumb and index finger can wrap around the base of his penis like a ring to keep things steady.

- Use your tongue to play along the ridge, the frenulum, the head of the penis, and all along the shaft while moving your mouth up and down his penis. It can take some coordination, but the key is really to relax, don't go *any* deeper than you are comfortable with, and have fun! Try to feel every square inch of his delicious manhood with the tip of your tongue.

- You can add the other hand to follow your lips either separately or as an extension of your mouth. Use your fingers in an okay sign or use your whole hand if he is larger or if you only want to have an inch or so of his penis in our mouth. Experiment with grip tension to see what he likes best. Some men prefer the same steady stroke, and others like you to change it up with different speeds, styles, and grip. Again, communication will work wonders.
- If he is uncircumcised, he will have a foreskin, which can act like a sleeve over the penis. It can be slid up and down, creating pleasure for him, and can be teased and played with by your tongue just as you would a circumcised man.
- Play and have fun!
- If you want to learn more, there are many great books about oral sex. I recommend Sadie Allison's *Tickle His Pickle*, which you can order from my Web site.

Orally Pleasing Your Woman

This is just for the men. Again, if you follow the guidelines in this chapter, are gentle with your woman, and communicate well, you can't go wrong. Most women love oral sex. The key to it is to tease her so she is practically begging you, and only then do you go for the clitoris. Many women have a hard time receiving pleasure and can start to feel guilty about it all being about them. The best thing you can do is to reassure her that you are in heaven when you go down on her and you love it, love it, love it!

- Make sure she is fully aroused before you even consider moving your mouth and tongue to her vulva and clitoris. She must be wet and turned on, or else she may push you away, since it isn't always pleasurable to have a mouth exploring between our legs when we aren't ready.

- Once you know she is all hot and rarin' to go, run your tongue and lips along her tummy, pausing for kisses or nibbles or whatever you've discovered she loves. Slowly make your way south.

- Then scoot around the area you most want to go to and lick, nibble, kiss, and tease her thighs all the way down to her knees. You should have her aching by now, and she may even grab your head to bring you close to her clitoris. If she does, go up there but then quickly move off somewhere else.

- When you've driven her mad, explore her vaginal opening with your tongue and all around her perineum. Some women enjoy a tongue darting into their vaginas; others like gentle vaginal lip nibbling. Experiment. (Be careful not to move your tongue near her anus if you plan to go back to the vaginal area, since she is more susceptible to infection from bacteria transfer.)

- When ready, go to her clitoris and enjoy. It should be harder now and will respond to your licking, tongue flicking, suckling, and finger rubbing. Some women like direct contact on the tip, and others like a back-and-forth motion on the side or at the base. For others, a circular motion while sucking directly, as though it were a small penis, is the most pleasurable. Think of the fun you will have discovering what her desire is.

- Once you start to build a rhythm and you can tell she is starting to get close to her orgasm, *don't stop what you are doing.* We like the pressure and pace to remain constant in order to reach orgasm, so don't speed up or do it harder unless she asks you to. Once she is climaxing, keep up the pace until she stops you—and she likely will—and revel in the fact that she is yours.

○ Play and have fun!
○ If you want to learn more, there are many great books about oral sex.

Deep Throat

Back to you, ladies! For a deeper oral sex experience, you need to adjust your throat position. Most women bend forward when loving their man's penis. When you do, your throat is bent and the penis can't get in very far. Instead, try lying on your back with your head dropping off the edge of the bed. Have your man standing before your tilted-back head and beckoning mouth. Grab his butt with your hands and be sure you are in charge of how deep he goes into your mouth. Arrange some signals in advance, since your mouth will be full!

Go slow, relax, and enjoy the amazement of your man as he watches you take more of him into your mouth than ever before. Even if you can't deep throat him, the sight of you laid out before him for his pleasure will be all he needs.

Decadent Accessories

Adding special ingredients to oral play is icing on an already delectable cake. Try any of these in your mouth to create cooling, warming, bubbling, or tingling sensations on your lover's privates. Try switching back and forth for titillating technique:

- Mints
- Mouthwash
- Cough drops
- Ice cubes
- Warm tea or water
- Pop Rocks candy
- Sparkling juice or water

Adding flavored treats is also delicious. Try whipped cream, chocolate or cherry sauce, icing sugar, or any other sticky sweetness. Be careful of pineapple or other acidic products that can cause stinging. Many a man has regretted having ring toss played with pineapple rings over his penis!

Be careful that none of these gets into the vagina as it will negatively impact the pH level. Using them up around the clitoris may be fine for some women. The safest bet for women are products designed specifically for oral sex so there are no sugars, which promote infection. But sweets for him are no problem. Bon appétit!

●●● Kim's **QUICKIE TIP**

Ice cream cones can be great foreplay. Practice slurping and swirling your tongue around a melting ice cream cone in front of your lover while pretending it is his yummy organ you are devouring. Use long, slow strokes of your tongue and then quick kitty-cat licks to start him melting.

A Prop or Two

Toys can add a range of sensations to the oral sex encounter. You can lick your lover's penis while he is being stimulated with a vibrating cock ring at the base or you can hold a regular vibrator at his frenulum (see diagram in chapter 3) while you lick around it. Suck on him while you toy with his testicles with a vibrator or have one on your cheek to make your mouth vibrate. If there is no toy available, try humming your favorite song or the national anthem (which will pass the vibrations along to him) and watch him stand at attention.

Keep the loving of your lover's loins a slippery affair. Unless you can provide copious quantities of saliva naturally, have a water-soluble, flavored lubricant handy to add the glide element that is a key to successful oral play.

Some tips and things to avoid regarding the penis:

Penis No-no's:
- Never compare it to any other penis.
- Don't scratch it (unless you're being very gentle and you know the penis well).
- Don't bite it (see previous bullet point).
- Don't grab it like a stick shift in a race car.
- Don't put rough hands on it (use lotion first so they are smooth).
- Don't put cold hands on it (rub them together first).
- Don't let your mouth or hands play with it if they are dry, unless you can glide easily without pulling.

Vulva No-no's:
All of the above, plus:
- Don't poke at it.
- Don't blow into the vagina.
- Don't dive onto the clitoris unless the lady is warmed up and ready.

The Eternal Question

The question of whether to spit or swallow your man's ejaculate is a personal one and only you can answer it. Your answer may change over time and in different circumstances. One or even many bad experiences in the past shouldn't be the only criteria you use. There are some options, though. Whatever you do, don't spit and gag and say how gross it is. You wouldn't want him to say that about your love juices!

You can have a cloth or towel handy and discreetly spit into it and continue touching and caressing him. Alternatively, if your head is bent over, let his semen slowly dribble out the corners of your mouth down along his penis. You don't have to swallow it just because it's in your mouth. Or when you realize he's about to orgasm, finish him off with your hand and maybe lick him along the shaft, his testicles, or his belly. How could he complain?

Oral Sex Shake Recipe

Yummy man, here you come! This sexy shake is a delicious recipe to make for your man so he'll be lip-smacking good for you during oral sex:

- 1 scoop natural vanilla ice cream
- Honey or sugar to sweeten
- 1 cup milk (or soy milk or rice milk)
- 1 pinch of any or all of the following dry spices: cardamom, allspice, cinnamon, ginger, cloves, or nutmeg
- ¼ cup diced pineapple
- 1 raw egg (optional—verify with your healthcare provider)

Blend all ingredients together in a blender. Serve one hour before lovemaking and his ejaculate will taste sweeter! I say you get bonus points if:

- you make this sexy shake yourself
- you feed it to him
- you spend the next hour massaging each other

Start your oral occurrences with a bang!

Condoms

Value yourself and your partner by practicing safe sex. Unless you are in a monogamous, committed relationship and have clean test results for sexually transmitted infections and diseases, condoms are a must. Learn how to roll one on with your mouth!

●●● Kim's **QUICKIE TIP**

In order to control your gag reflex, you can put some numbing gel on the back of your tongue. Use the same gels designed for teething babies or Kama Sutra's Pleasure Balm Desensitizing Gel (which you can find on my Web site, www.kimswitnicki.com/greatsexforhardtimes).

Consider the condom a loving part of your union. Your mind-set will make all the difference. Incorporate condom play into your bedroom so it becomes an automatic, necessary, and fun part of your sex play.

SEXY CHALLENGE
Sweet Torture

You'll Need: Both of your bodies
Prep Time: None
Cost: $0
Raciness Factor: Bold
Benefit: Improves Sexual Skills

Start at one of your man's knees and take ten minutes to slowly go all the way up to his lips, bypassing the genitals entirely. Use at least three different strokes, nibbles, kisses, or gentle scratches to get there. Then start down at the other knee. The torture will be sweet, and you can reward him with a delicious French kiss on his penis and take it anywhere you like from there!

chapter 14

Food and Sex—Lovemaking Recipes to Satisfy All Your Cravings

Your words are my food, your breath my wine. You are everything to me. —**Sarah Bernhardt, actress**

Food can add mouthwatering excitement to your sex play. Sex and food have been bosom buddies for centuries. Going back in time, Roman orgies involving nude servants and feasts of sumptuous delight were commonplace. High-society dinner parties attended by decadent royalty and mistresses alike enjoyed nude dining on caviar, quail, and marzipan. Before the French Revolution, some restaurants did double duty as brothels and provided digestive aids in the form of nude dancers performing among the tables.

Aphrodisiacs in the food world are many. There are foods purported to have direct libido-boosting properties due to their shape, seductiveness, and suggestive power both when eaten or during preparation. Have you ever looked closely at a papaya split in half? Or at an asparagus stalk as a woman slowly inserts it between her red lips, Béarnaise sauce dripping out of the corner of her mouth as her tongue darts out and seductively scoops it up? Some foods are phallic, like asparagus and bananas, or resemble the vulva, such as oysters, peaches, figs, or papaya. Can you think of any others?

Sensual Feast

Since *sensual* means "of the senses," be sure to incorporate more than taste into your evening. Visual displays of foods with tasty textures and aromatic bouquets to tempt the palette are powerful elements of sensual affairs. Think soft, bubbly, and slippery. Savor the textures of cuisine, such as the softness of fresh raspberries as they roll around on your lover's tummy, the fluffy frothiness of whipped cream as you lick it off his chest, the bubbliness of champagne as you share a kiss after a mouthful, or the slipperiness of a mango or a peach as you prepare slices to hand-feed your man.

Aroma alone can be a stimulating aphrodisiac. Men have been known to be aroused by pumpkin pie spices or the aroma of vanilla, while women are known to respond to licorice and cucumber. Smells zoom right to the emotional center of your brain before any other sensory stimuli. Use this to your advantage and encompass multiple fragrances into love play and be thankful you aren't a goat. The male goat will often urinate and ejaculate into his beard, using his pungent odor to show off his masculinity to female suitors!

Kinky Kitchen

One of the most popular mainstream sex scenes of modern times is the "fridge scene" in the film *9½ Weeks* with Mickey Rourke and Kim Basinger. The sense of excitement, mystery, anticipation, and blind trust she puts in him is palpable as he teases her mouth with unknown foods (her eyes are closed) while they sit on the floor, lit by only the fridge bulb. He unleashes cherries, honey, and a green chili pepper onto her tongue and then lets her wash it all down with milk in a finale that is very hot indeed. If you haven't seen this movie, it's definitely worth renting for some inspiration.

When, Where, and How

First things first, you need to entice your lover to come to the table or wherever you plan to serve your meal. Any of these following ideas are sure to capture his attention, win his heart, and create memorable moments for your mental scrapbook of romance:

- Present him with a list of appetizers, entrées, and desserts that you know he loves and have him circle one from each category with a bright red lipstick.

- Provide a pair of panties with a handwritten invitation (in dollar-store lipstick) sprayed with your favorite perfume and tucked into an envelope. Be sure to add that he is to shower before dinner. Mail them a week in advance, pop them in his briefcase, or leave them on the seat of his car so he finds them on his way to work. Build the anticipation!

- Use a steamy shower mirror to write him a message letting him know what time dinner is and not to be late. Say the kids will be at a friend's if that helps (arrange this in advance).

○ Leave silky stockings, a bra, and panties with a pair of your sexiest shoes on the bathroom counter so he sees them when he gets out of the shower. Tuck the invitation inside a shoe.

Recipe Ideas for Passionate Feasts

After you've decided how you plan to lure your lover and the destination, you can start working on the menu and what you'll be serving. There are various foods to choose from, and here are a few recipes you might enjoy preparing.

Oysters

It has been said that Casanova indulged in oysters for breakfast. Their slurp factor, which some find repugnant, can be highly erotic. Known as "seaducers" they may be aphrodisiacal because they can change their sex for reproduction purposes. Kinky devils!

Don't forget that you yourself are a feast for the eyes. While you feed your lover some fresh oysters, be sure to slowly undress while whispering how slippery and sensual they must feel on his tongue. Remove one button after each oyster or hike up your skirt a little higher with each scrumptious mouthful!

Asparagus and Papaya

You've likely heard the cliché "The way to a man's heart is through his stomach," and it's true. A candlelit meal is a surefire romance starter. Your thoughtfulness will not go unnoticed or unrewarded. Candlelight is very flattering and allows you to stare deeply into each others' eyes. Dress the part of the seductress, or serving wench if you prefer, and offer a banquet he can't wait to devour. Drip warm butter over fresh asparagus as you serve it to him. Engage his erotic desire by s-l-o-w-l-y slurping entire stems of asparagus. Watch him melt as you lick the butter off of each piece.

For dessert, slice open a papaya and feed small, soft, silky slices to him by hand. One for him, one for you, one for him, and what comes next?

●●● Kim's **QUICKIE TIP**

No utensils allowed when feeding your lover. Simply lick each other's fingers for erotic visions of what is to come. . . .

Grapes and Cucumber

Wearing an apron, heels, and a smile, greet your man when he comes home from a hard day at work. Things can only go up from here! Invite him to join you in the shower. Have seedless grapes waiting and ready to drop into his mouth whenever he speaks. He'll catch on soon that this is a silent affair (except for the moaning to come). After you've cleaned each other and gotten each other sufficiently hot, bring out the surprise—a cucumber. Wash it as you wash his penis and feel how hard they both are. Whisper that you've always wanted two men at once and this is a way to fulfill your fantasy. Make sure you have lots of lubricant and decide ahead of time whether you want the cucumber inside your vagina or you want to play anally, and guide him along. Hang on tight and enjoy the ride!

●●● Kim's **QUICKIE TIP**

Share food prep, such as cutting up veggies or marinating meat, with a passionate kiss in between each activity.

SEXY CHALLENGE
Passion Picnic

You'll Need: Picnic location, music, food, perfume
Prep Time: 2+ hours
Cost: $20+ (depending on your choices)
Raciness Factor: Bold
Benefit: Develops Intimacy

Prepare a passion picnic. Select a location and be adventurous. Options: your bed, your bedroom floor, your living room floor, a tent, your backyard, a beach, by a lake, a friends' yard, or a friends' house. Add romantic lighting and music if you can to calm and relax you. Prepare some of his favorite foods and something delicious he enjoys drinking. This will show him you are devoted to all his pleasures. Wear his favorite scent and do your hair the way he likes. Remember to lick his fingers and anything else that comes up.

Zucchini and Carrots? Yes!

Much has been said (all good!) about slightly microwaved zucchini or carrots. They may be rubbery to eat, but mild cooking can render them as fabulous dildos. Smooth-shaped vegetables such as cucumbers, carrots, and zucchini lend themselves well to this quest. The thrill of being naughty may also add to the allure of veggie sex play. Experiment ahead of time with different veggies and your microwave so you can be well prepared. Ask him if he would be interested in a new erotic veggie dip you read about. Take his hand and let him know you are the dipping bowl while you lead him to your bedroom, all set up with veggies, lubricant, and mood lighting for a night of decadent playtime.

●●● Kim's **QUICKIE TIP**

Carrots are especially nice as anal toys because they start small and get bigger. Be careful, be safe, and have fun!

Chocolate Mousse and Whipped Cream

If you don't want to dine naked, at least clean up after dinner in the nude. Make a show of removing your clothes and his and then take him up to the bathtub. Wash yourselves and let him know you'll be right back with dessert. Hop out of the tub and come back with chocolate mousse and a can of whipped cream. Hand-feed each other the mousse in the bathtub. In between each fingerful, draw a name or heart or other symbol on each other with the whipped cream and then lick off every last bit. Toss in some bubbles, candles, and sparkling juice and you have heaven for two. Or add the special cordial (recipe on page 186) mixed with white wine or sparkling water for some erotic flair.

Violet Delight

It has been said that violets were a common ingredient in love potions and were thought to be the plant of ancient goddesses and a symbol of love and faithfulness. They make the skin glow, provide a glorious aftertaste, and help us feel happy. Here is a recipe for a violet cordial for you to create your own love potion for passion:

- 2 cups spring water
- About ½ pound fresh, organic violets, separated
- 2 cups honey
- Egg whites
- Sugar
- White wine or sparkling water

Put eight violets aside for crystallizing. Boil the spring water and pour over remaining violets. Cover and let cool. Steep overnight in a ceramic dish. The next day, strain out the flowers. Add the violet water to the honey in a heavy saucepan. Gently bring to a boil and simmer for fifteen to twenty minutes or until syrupy. Cool and pour into a clean jar and keep refrigerated. On the special day, take the violets you put aside, brush both sides in egg whites, dredge them in sugar, and let them dry on waxed paper. Pour a shot of the syrupy cordial into frosted glasses, add white wine or sparkling water, and place the crystallized violets on top of each glass. Serve immediately and let your passion bloom!

Strawberries and Sweet Delights

Cultivate your creativity muscle by practicing feeding your lover using a variety of your curvaceous body parts. Make sure you're clean, of course, and pass strawberries to his lips using your toes (especially if he has a foot fetish), proffer sweet syrups from your breasts, or present him chocolate kisses nestled in your under-arms. What other hands-free offerings can you create?

Bananas *(Wink, wink . . .)*

Satisfy your craving for sweets by enjoying a banana split with your lover's penis as the centerpiece. Layer whipped cream and chocolate sauce or swirl both around his penis like a barber's pole and place a cherry on top. Add some sprinkles and watch his eyes get bigger and bigger as his anticipation builds. Lick it off as slowly as possible to drive him to the edge and back. **Note:** Be sure to have the penis licked off or washed before vaginal penetration.

I Scream for Ice Cream

Eating or feeding each other in the nude not only is fun but feels exotic, decadent, and somehow animalistic. Just watch out for hot sauces, gravies, or dips. Colder fare such as ice cream begs to be spilled onto you. Jen's first sexy food experience ensured it won't be her last:

> We were enjoying a wickedly romantic evening on our big picnic blanket, which I spread out on the bed. The meal was seafood with sauces and asparagus. Who knew they went so well together? I had just delivered two ice cream cones and was seducing him by licking mine in all the right places. It was melting faster than I could keep up with, since I had the heat up in the room so we'd stay warm. Inevitably, it started dripping down the cone and

onto my breasts and thighs. I looked him in the eye with my best vixen stare and demanded he lean forward immediately and lick the ice cream off my breasts and thighs. Oh my, did he ever. Lionel was ravenous!

Luckily we still had a plate on the bed for the shrimp shells and our two cones promptly ended up on that plate. We made a bit of a sticky mess, but the blanket washed up and so did we!

Let food set the stage for your next sensual encounter. While these foods are seductive in appearance, they may not actually boost your libido. However, they *can* inspire you to switch from dinner to dessert in a hurry or to combine both for mouthwatering delights.

Food Fight

Yoko and Jim have been known to start the odd food fight with mini tomatoes ricocheting through the kitchen and frozen peas spit out of straws, only to be found behind the stove a month later! Yoko finds that getting playful with Jim is what she needs at the end of a long day:

We love to horse around. It can break up the tension of the day, and the laughter keeps me grounded and connected to home, shutting the troubles of the outside world away.

Go ahead and have fun with your food and with each other—genuine intimacy can and often does lead to better sex.

Natural Sex Toys

When funds are tight for dildos or you simply want to investigate the idea of using food as a novelty sex toy, a few words of caution. We live in an age of pesticides, herbicides, and other chemicals on our food to "protect" us from harm, and these substances are not designed for the vagina. Wash thoroughly or, better yet, apply a condom on any item being inserted into a vagina or anus. As long as you are both consenting and having a good time, it's all perfectly healthy and normal, so enjoy the possibilities!

SEXY CHALLENGE
Bodacious Body Art

You'll Need: Fresh fruit, sauces, sprinkles, nuts, candles, music, a robe or towel, a camera
Prep Time: 1+ hour
Cost: $20+
Raciness Factor: Bold
Benefit: Develops Intimacy

Turn your lover into a sculpture of decadence. Prepare bowls of fresh sliced fruit (strawberries, kiwis, grapes, melons, and bananas), some delicious sauces (chocolate, fresh whipped cream, mousse, yogurt, or pudding), and some candied or chocolate sprinkles with slivers of almonds or sunflower seeds.

Take a sensuous bubble bath, then lead him to a warmed-up room with scented candles and mood music. Disrobe him slowly (or unwrap him from a towel) after patting him dry and lay him down gently, kissing him from head to toe as you whisper how much you love and cherish each part of him and all he does for

you. Start to adorn his body with the ingredients you have prepared. Take a picture when you're done as a souvenir.

Option: If you're an artist, sketch him, or else take a short
video from his head to his sexy toes.

When we were younger we were told not to play with our food,
but allow me to give you complete and total permission to play
with your food and your partner. The next time you pick up
groceries, consider adding a few of these sexy foods to your
cart—they will help get you and your hottie in the mood:

- Oysters
- Asparagus
- Papaya
- Cucumbers
- Grapes
- Zucchini
- Carrots
- Chocolate
- Whipped cream
- Strawberries
- Bananas
- Ice cream
- Chocolate sauce
- Figs
- Raspberries
- Truffles
- Avocado

chapter 15

Waterfalls, Hot Tubs, Showers, and More To Keep You Hot, Wet, and Ready

You don't need to be on the same wavelength to succeed in marriage. You just need to be able to ride each other's waves.

—Toni Sciarra Poynter, author, *This Day Forward: Meditations on the First Years of Marriage*

Imagine the excitement of a waterfall rushing over your naked body. Now picture yourself with your lover, enjoying the headiness of swimming naked in a river, ocean, or lake. Imagine you are the carefree and wild Aphrodite—a goddess of love born from the foam of the sea. Water has always had a mythical place in the annals of love. How can you make your own wet dreams real? What follows are some ideas to help you do just that.

Birthday Treat

Yoko surprised her hubby with this treat for his summertime birthday. You'll score points with this too, no matter what type of vehicle you have, but it is especially effective if your man loves his car.

Luckily it happened that the kids were off at camp the week of Jim's birthday. I arose early, set his alarm to go off in an hour, and left a little note saying coffee was ready and to join me in the driveway. I put on some sweet, short shorts and a white tank top, set the coffeemaker for fifty minutes, and prepared a bucket of hot, soapy water. I then grabbed the sponges and chamois and went out and washed our company truck until it sparkled. I had it all rinsed off and was halfway through drying it when I noticed the time was getting tight.

Racing back into the house, I rinsed out the bucket and filled it with warm water as I inhaled the aroma of fresh brewed coffee. Back outside I went with my refilled bucket. I draped myself along the hood of the truck in what I hoped was a seductive pose and waited for my man to appear. I was enjoying the heat of the morning sun on my body, drying up my clothes right away. Jim appeared at the top of the driveway looking sleepy, sipping his steaming mug of coffee. His eyes went big as saucers as he watched me pick up a sponge from the bucket (sitting on a towel behind me so I didn't scratch the paint on the hood), hold it over my head, and squeeze so the warm water swooshed down my arms and all over my lovely white tank top.

I'll let you imagine the rest from there. Let's just say his coffee got cold, and every time he drives the truck, he has a hot memory to make him smile.

💜 Please be aware of laws regarding public nudity where you live. The risk is enticing and has added many titillating memories for yours truly, but safety is paramount.

●●● Kim's **QUICKIE TIP**

Start your day with a stimulating (minty, tingly, or spicy) shower gel to wake up your skin and your other senses, and to add zest to your day.

Be Lubed

Enter when wet. This is the golden rule for penetration, and for water play you need to be especially prepared. Just because you have water around you (in the shower or tub, for example) and your vagina feels wet, you may not be sufficiently lubricated enough for the insertion of a finger, toy, or penis. Slipperiness is essential, so be prepared with a lubricant to make sure you have a satisfying bout.

There are pros and cons to all types of lubricants. Here are the basics:

Water-soluble lubricants are nonstaining, nonirritating, and wash away quickly with water. This is fabulous in the bedroom because it comes off and out of you easily, so there is no risk of bacteria developing internally.

You never want to use an oil-based lubricant, because oil can stay in your body for up to three days, creating a breeding ground for bacteria. Plus, oil breaks down latex. Condom compatibility may be important to you, so oils are a no-no.

Silicone-based lubricants are the most slippery, but won't wash away easily, so they are a great addition to water play. Be aware that these may stay inside your vagina longer than the water-soluble options. **Note:** Don't buy a lubricant containing nonoxynol-9, since it may irritate sensitive vaginal tissue, promoting the spread of infection or HIV.

●●● Kim's **QUICKIE TIP**

If your lubricant is getting sticky, the water has evaporated from it. Reconstitute it with a spritz of water—on you, not in the bottle—to juicy it up again. Keep a water pistol by the bed for fun!

Hot Tub Love

While lubricant is important, a location for water play is an important factor as well. Sizzling hot-tub sex is a common fantasy. The reality is that intercourse is not advised while in a hot tub. The hot water and chemicals will quickly sluice away your natural lubricant, so you may more easily tear on penetration. It will be hard not to notice you are technically "dry" or unprotected for penetration. The chemicals can irritate the sensitive vaginal lining and bacteria can get a foothold and breed. *Sex play should be kept above the water line.* If you decide to indulge and you are using a super-slippery silicone (or any other) lubricant, all surfaces it touches will become dangerous, especially when you add water, since it may juice itself up even further!

Be careful of water getting pushed into the vagina when the penis is inserted. This may be uncomfortable and potentially dangerous for the woman and may also push irritants, such as chemicals or bacteria, inside her. This also applies to sex in oceans, rivers, and lakes.

No matter what anyone says, yes, you *can* get pregnant in a hot tub!

Shower Love

Another popular location for steaming it up is in the shower. The Shower Steam position in chapter 9 is an example of a sultry pose for the shower. If you have a soap holder, use it as a handy place to grip while lovemaking under the spray. Leaning forward with your hands against the wall, offering your rear for your lover to snuggle in close to, is a favorite position for shower love.

Beware if you are hopping into the shower to clean up after loving, because as soon as the water stream hits your body, residue from lubricant will rinse right off you and onto the floor of the tub. A shower mat is a good idea for getting a grip when lubricants may make the tub slippery.

Also consider adding natural steam to your man's shower by surprising him and hopping in to join him when he isn't expecting it. After all, you can never be too clean. If he likes to take baths, bend over and give him a super-passionate kiss and let him pull you in (with a little prompting if needed), clothes and all!

💜 Shower loving is perfect during your period. Mess? What mess? Women are generally hornier during their periods, and sex has been known to reduce cramping too!

Water Toys

Once you're in a slippery spot, you may want to add a toy that is a little more fun than a plain old rubber duckie. I'm often asked if there are special waterproof toys for water play. While most "waterproof" toys are in fact water resistant and not waterproof, no harm will come to you if you drop them in the tub or get them wet. They'll simply stop. While inconvenient, it isn't disastrous. *Do not* use plug-in toys near water.

A truly fun toy is a dong that has a suction cup on the base so you can stick it to the wall of your shower or even the floor. Bend down and squat over it or bend forward and back into it slowly. I offer a lovely purple one on my Web site. The beauty of using it anally is that washup is a cinch! Whether you are alone or with your man, this can be a decadent sensation. You might consider simulating a fantasy of two men at a time without the potential pitfalls and with all of the satisfaction.

My favorite G-spot vibrator is waterproof, as are lots of other vibrators.

Water Games and Books

You can also add entertainment to hot tubs, baths, and Jacuzzis with water games such as Bathtub Love, which is a set of plastic eggs containing waterproof sexy suggestions for things to do in the tub. There are waterproof love dice, for a game in which every roll's a winner, and even a vibrating rubber duckie! Check my Web site at www.kimswitnicki.com/greatsexforhardtimes to see all of my sexy offerings.

Allow your sense of adventure out to play with the Aqua Erotica books. They're perfect for the bath or even the shower because they are *waterproof books*! They are the best I've seen so far. Not only are they hot and sexy, covering all sorts of wicked and wonderful situations, but the fact that you can get them wet is just what the doctor ordered. The first in the series contains stories that all have an element of water in them. The second isn't water-based, but gets into the kinkier side of fantasy and will help you bust your inhibitions and discover more of what really makes your erotic engine tick. I keep one on our boat so that when the mood strikes, I'm ready! Perhaps by this printing there will be a third. If so, it will be available on my Web site as well.

SEXY CHALLENGE
Tropical Delight

You'll Need: A robe or towel, a dryer, shampoo, a water jug, candles, sparkling juice, music, a warm room, tropical-scented massage oil
Prep Time: 10 minutes
Cost: $0–$10
Raciness Factor: Regular
Benefit: Develops Intimacy

Pop a robe (or towel) into the dryer to get it toasty warm while you sensuously bathe your lover. Wash his hair using a jug or container to rinse the shampoo, stand him up, and admire him as you wash each body part slowly and sensuously. Lick the water off of him and then rinse him with warm fresh water. When finished, invite him to relax, light some more candles, and hand him a glass of sparkling juice and go get the warm robe (or towel), fresh out of the dryer. Help him out of the tub, pat him dry with a clean towel (or the warmed-up one) and wrap him in the robe (or the towel). Now you are ready to lay him down on your bed in a room you warmed up ahead of time. Invite him to imagine being on a tropical beach (add beach music with waves if you can). Apply coconut or mango massage oil to his warmed body. You can take it from here.

$ $ $ Kim's **CASH SAVER**

Dollar stores often have inexpensive small bottles of massage oils. They may not last long, but once is enough!

SEXY CHALLENGE
Exotic Treat for Two

You'll Need: An invitation (can be a simple handwritten note), plants, scented candles, paper umbrellas, fruit juice, bathing suits (his and hers), a beach towel, blue food coloring (safe for fabrics), simple finger foods

Optional: A bamboo screen, a beach mat, beach towels, sandals, tropical flowers, a beach ball, fresh tropical fruits (pineapple, mango, bananas, papaya, coconut), a Waterpik for self-stimulation in the tub, a massaging showerhead, a rainfall showerhead, sand and a plastic sheet or tarp, a hula skirt, a Hawaiian lei

Prep Time: 30 minutes to 2 hours, depending on how extravagant the scene

Cost: $0–$100

Raciness Factor: Extreme

Benefit: Increases Inner Sensuality

Create a tropical haven in your bathroom and plan a romantic getaway for two. Hang a beach towel with a tropical scene over your bathroom window so it looks like you have the beach or another exotic locale right outside. Serve your man tropical juice with a paper umbrella in it while you hand him his invitation to a tropical oasis for two. Toss him his bathing suit and a beach towel and have him join you in the bathroom. He walks in to discover you've turned your bathroom into an exotic oasis of sensual pleasures for the evening or afternoon. He can see plants throughout the room (most houseplants can handle some warm, moist air for a few hours) and the air is still steamy since you just turned off the shower, which was on (hot water only) for about ten minutes. The exotic scent of the candles infuses everything with tropical aromas. He spies the platter of simple yet erotic foods and a pitcher of fresh juice to quench his upcoming thirst, and you rejoice in the smile spreading across his face!

You can get in the blue water in the tub you prepared in advance (yes, using some of the water while running the shower earlier) with your suits on or off. Start by showing him how you can please yourself using the Waterpik, a showerhead massager (if handheld), or the tub faucet to bring yourself to orgasm. (Try this on your own first so you know what to expect and to determine the most comfortable position! This can be a big turn-on for men who've heard of this mysterious activity but have rarely seen it.) Then hand-feed each other and enjoy what comes naturally in paradise.

To make it extraordinary, hang a fern or eucalyptus plant from the showerhead or install a rainfall showerhead (from a hardware or bathroom store) into your shower. If you have a rain-type option on your massager, that works too. Add as many of the optional items as you can, and more if you can think of any—have fun with it!

$ $ $ Kim's **CASH SAVER**

Dollar stores offers paper umbrellas, beach towels, beach mats, lovely paper or plastic flowers, sandals, and beach toys to add ambiance and playfulness to your sexy beach scene.

chapter **16**

Quickies in the Moment—Fast-Paced Sex for Today's Fast-Paced Couple

Remember, if you smoke after sex you're doing it too fast. —**Woody Allen, actor/director**

Hard kisses and strong embraces are the hallmarks of quickie sex. Take charge of the situation in the moment to help you let go of any anxiety around sex. "Harder," "faster," and "deeper" are the words to use. Coming on strong can be just what it takes to bring you both from zero to sixty in ten seconds or less. In the fast-paced lifestyle most of us find ourselves in, a quickie may be all we can squeeze in. So make it count!

When squeezing in a quick tumble, remember that orgasm should not be your only aim. In fact, orgasm shouldn't be the goal at any time. The actual act of linking together physically is often all you need for either one of you to de-stress after a bad day, decompress after bad news, get reconnected emotionally, or simply have some quick recreational fun!

On Getting to It

These days, time seems to be in short supply. Yet we want to feel connected to our mates, we have physical yearnings to satisfy, and we know (if we've read this far) that continuing to have great sex will help calm us and help us enjoy life so much more. To that end, what follows are some ideas for the many places and options you have for gratification for both of you.

Kitchen

- Kitchen tables are often just the right height for leaning onto and having your man spoon you from behind.
- Fulfill your waitress-gets-overtaken-by-an-excitable-customer fantasy by grabbing a pillow or a kitchen chair cushion to slip under you as you sprawl yourself out flat on your back on the table.
- If you sit up on the table or counter, you can grab his shirt and hang on tight as he enters you right from the edge.
- Pretend you're in a sizzling sex scene in a movie and lean over the kitchen counter or hop onto it and offer up your sweet treats to your man.

Office (Home or Business) and Quiet Little Corners

Consider dressing in high heels, stockings, a short skirt, and whatever else you fancy, all hidden under a trench coat. Even one of his big coats will do. As long as you're completely covered up except for your sexy shoes. Walk down the driveway like this to meet your man after work. Or meet him like this if you have to pick him up from the airport after a trip. Maybe you're just meeting somewhere in the middle of the day and only have thirty minutes together. Whatever the reason, make it worth both your whiles by driving him wild with desire for you and what you have under your coat.

You can also send a quick e-mail or a text, or call him, asking, "Your office or mine?"—which is bound to get any man's heart pumping. Make sure you greet him wearing your trench coat. The library can be a sweet spot for a quiet make-out session if you go to a seldom-used section. A trench coat may work here also—just don't get caught by the librarian!

Stairway (or Elevator) to Heaven

Passion can be easily found in an elevator (remember the elevator scene in *Fatal Attraction*?) or on a stairway. Use these functional locations for more than getting from point A to point B, unless A is for amorous and B is for bold. Stairwells aren't just for the movies either. Exciting events with stockings bared, skirts hiked, and lips locked are perfect for a rarely used landing between flights of stairs.

Getting Away

Absence can certainly make the heart grow fonder. Being apart for a little while is good for any relationship, and a pending absence is a great excuse for a quickie. Staying over at a friend's place or taking a short trip to see relatives is an opportunity for a frantic fool-around either in the car before you go or the night you come home. Make this scenario a devilish role play and pretend you haven't seen each other for weeks to speed things up while you rush to get each other undressed.

Midnight Merriment

Sometimes a midnight quickie is necessary, especially if you want to take your man by surprise in an oh-you-wicked-girl way.

Jen surprised Lionel in the middle of the night:

We hadn't been making love a whole lot and I wanted to get some of our old spark back. I often get up at least once in the night. This particular evening I had been having a rather erotic dream and was disappointed to wake up before things got really hot. I went to use the bathroom like usual. On my way back to bed, I stopped at the door. I stood admiring my handsome husband, whose face was glowing from a half-moon shining through the window. His brow was so relaxed in sleep and he looked so peaceful. I was filled with warmth and a rush of love for this man who tried so hard to provide all he could for me and our two kids.

I quietly opened my closet door and slipped a long purple negligee off a hanger in the far corner. It had been a Valentine's Day gift from my sweet husband, and I'd hardly worn it. I pulled my plain old nightgown over my head, dropped it at my feet, and slipped the soft, silky negligee on. It's amazing how I can feel instantly prettier, younger, and sexier when I wear it!

I padded over to Lionel's side of the bed and pulled the sheet back down off his shoulder. I knelt down on the floor and leaned over, kissing his shoulder blades, his neck, and the top of his arm. He was smooth and warm and his scent made my belly tingle with the beginnings of desire. He stirred and made a soft sound but remained asleep. My hand slid down his back and over his butt and down between his legs. One leg was up, so I had room to caress and tease his balls and squeeze his thigh. He instinctively re-

acted by squeezing his butt cheeks and pressing himself into the mattress. I felt myself getting wet.

I slowly rolled him over, using his bent leg as leverage. He allowed me to move him whichever way I wanted. I wasn't sure if he was really asleep, but that didn't matter. When he was on his back, my mouth found his belly and I kissed my way down to his penis, which was surprisingly hard at this point. I moved him over to the middle of the bed a bit more so I could squat down over him with a leg on either side. I leaned forward and started nuzzling his neck with my lips. At that his hands woke up (if not the rest of him), and they both came up to my waist. As he felt the silky material, he moaned. Or maybe it was then that I lowered my moistened self down onto his erection. I slid on easily and lowered myself right down to the base of his penis. He said my name, which made me swoon, and we made love quickly but intently with both of us climaxing within minutes.

When it was over, I reached into his bedside table drawer for a wipe that he keeps handy and then snuggled him back under the sheet, and he was right back asleep. I got up to wash and noticed a huge smile on my face as I glanced in the mirror on my way back to bed. "You go girl!" I said to my reflection. I've finally found the switch inside me to make my own sparks fly.

In the morning, Lionel shared with all of us at break-fast that he had the best sleep ever as he winked at me. I think I blushed!

Note: Be sure you're aroused, so you're wet and your vagina and other organs have had time to shift into optimal position for penetration, or else you may find intercourse uncomfortable. Read on further for tips to speed up this process.

Sneaking Kisses with Kids Around

Having kids around can put the squeeze on lover time. Look around your house with fresh eyes for the great places to connect, even when the kids are in the house. Do you have a private outdoor patio or balcony suitable for romance? A laundry room (with the washer operating to cover up any sounds) can be warm and exciting enough to keep you spinning. Lean against the washer during the spin cycle for vibrations to enhance the experience. Juanita enjoys the shower for couples time. Yoko says she and Jim sneak kisses and lustily grab at each other in the hallway as foreplay for the coming night. Dear friends of mine have a huge walk-in closet that suits them perfectly for a morning tryst while they get ready for work. Jen says the car is one of her favorite places to escape for some making out:

> *Lionel and I got together in college and I lived on campus in girls-only dorms, so we didn't have too many places to go. His roommates were always around, so we ended up in the car most nights we were together. His kisses have improved over the years, and he knows all the places to touch me.*
>
> *We have a minivan, and sometimes after we drop the kids at soccer or hockey practice (we go to all their games, though), he'll reach for me in the parking lot. We hop onto the bench seat in the back and make out. It takes me back to our college days, and even now we steam up the windows!*

Car sex can be uncomfortable, but Jen has found that the bench seat works great for her. Some cars have extra head room. That sounds like an invitation for fun if I ever heard one!

She Made Me Do It

What would your man do if you walked up to him wearing a man's dress shirt and a pair of bikini undies, planted a 10-Second Kiss on him (see chapter 6), and then whispered huskily in his ear, "Tear it off me, big boy," while his hands were wandering all over your body?

Wet Love

Add spark to his engine by hopping in the shower with him while wearing your man's dress shirt and then tear the shirt off yourself. It won't be only the buttons flying high!

$ $ $ Kim's **CASH SAVER**

Pick up a man's oversized dress shirt at a local thrift store to tear off yourself.

Having a Solid Base

If you have active, small children, you may be simply too tired to have sex. As long as you keep the lines of communication open, maintain intimacy, and have a solid foundation of love and friendship in your marriage, you'll be fine. Don't get hung up feeling that you must have sex if it isn't going to work out for you to do it right at that moment. Make sure you are both on the same page, though, so one of you isn't feeling left out. The little things, like regular 10-Second Kisses, lunch or dinner dates, and walks around the neighborhood holding hands are all good to keep you connected while you weather the joys and trials of small children.

Just a Taste

Oral and manual play are glorious alternatives to full-out intercourse. Sometimes you don't feel like the whole enchilada. Treat each other or just please your partner. What a wonderful way to maintain intimacy without rejection. Just be sure you are 100 percent committed, so the contact is authentic. You may just want to "help out" your partner by whispering sexy things in his ear or playing with his nipples or testicles while he plays with himself. This can be a powerful, intimate way to express your love for him. He's sure to appreciate it!

Make-Up Quickies

Some couples don't mean to have quickies, but they find that a hard-and-fast session of make-up sex can be intense, aggressive (in a good way), and oh-so-wonderful. Michelle and Dave had never had sex after a fight before:

> With my recent attention to my sexuality and stirring the pot of my libido, I found out that arguing actually got me hot! Dave and I had gotten into a big fight. I can't remember what it was even about, but there was yelling and cursing and slamming of doors. I finally went up to him and got right in his face, saying that if he didn't shut up, I'd make him. He looked me in the eyes and said, "Make me," real quiet-like.
>
> I can't believe I did this, but I grabbed him with both hands on the sides of his head and kissed him—hard! It took him a bit, but soon he started kissing me back. Well! Our clothes ended up strewn all over the living room as we tore them off ourselves on our way to the bedroom. We were like animals. By the time we got to the act, I was even a

bit wet. I paused him before he went inside me, just so I
could put a bit more lube on, but then off we went. It was
incredible!

Create Anticipation

Romance is another secret to a long and strong marriage. Build the anticipation for as long as possible ahead of time so the quickie becomes the culmination of hours or even days of foreplay. Tease each other with flirting looks, steamy kisses, and suggestive caresses all day or even all week. This works especially well if you find you are tired or don't have much time, and is also a great way to let your lover know you desire him. This extended foreplay will be your guarantee that your body will be more than ready for the next encounter, even if it is a quickie.

Some people don't like the idea of setting appointments for love because they feel it is unromantic. Think of it as building the intensity in advance. Anticipating upcoming lovemaking is a powerful aphrodisiac. When we first met our lovers, we invariably made dates, which were actually appointments for lovemaking in some cases! Not always, but in most cases we dressed and waxed and washed and styled and primped ourselves for what we hoped would be a hot time, right? Make these dates no different.

Getting in Sync

You might find that, between the two of you, it seems your timing is off and you aren't both available for sex at the same time. Or you aren't feeling frisky at the same time. Try this if that is the case: Observe when you find yourself aroused. Chart on a simple piece of paper all the times when you're in the mood for three weeks. This is useful for both of you to do. Afterward, look at both charts to see if there are any patterns. You may find that after a workout you're both turned on. If you work out on different days, that doesn't do much for your sex life. If this is an area you can modify so you're both aroused at the same time, go for it!

Your charts may show other patterns that can help you fine-tune your schedules so you're in the same place, physically and mentally ready for love. Attention to your patterns may be all you need to increase the quickie factor in your life.

Get in the Mood First

We've determined that anticipation is a great way of preparing yourself in advance so you're ready for a sexy quickie. You can also use fantasy to your advantage. Daydream in the car—keep your eyes on the road!—or on a coffee break or while making your lunch, doing some shopping, or, my favorite, in the bathtub. If you get yourself into a frenzy of lust fantasizing about whatever in the world works to get you hot, and you hunt down your man for a fast and furious frolic, no one will complain!

Another tried-and-true way to get some women's juices flowing is to write, read, or watch erotica. Try any or all of them for expanding your repertoire of sexy images to use for self-stimulation. Erotica in any form is a useful accessory for the two of you to enjoy together.

SEXY CHALLENGE
Come Catch Me

You'll Need: The two of you
Prep Time: None
Cost: $0
Raciness Factor: Bold
Benefit: Increases Inner Sensuality

Play chase with each other and work up a good sweat. This rowdy workout will get your endorphins going and boost your chances for a sweaty encounter. Wrestle him to the ground, sit on top of him, and lean in for a hard kiss while you take his hand and help him squeeze your breast. This may never be an Olympic sport, but practice like it is!

$ $ $ Kim's **CASH SAVER**

Chase each other indoors or out with dollar-store squirt guns, making a wet kiss the "penalty" for getting hit.

chapter **17**

Sizzling Sex Adventures—From Learning Pole Dancing to Setting Up Safe Threesomes

It does not matter what you do in the bedroom as long as you do not do it in the street and frighten the horses. —**Mrs. Patrick Campbell, actress**

Sex adventures dress up a ho-hum sex life like nothing else. Putting time and attention into your love life is crucial to keeping it vibrant and alive. What better way to maintain and improve things in the bedroom than with some escapades?

If you want to keep your man, then keep him entertained by being unpredictable and surprise him with unexpected bedroom behavior. Consider entertaining his fantasies and you can be sure he will reward you with lots of loyalty, love, and great lovin'.

In this chapter I explore a variety of sexual adventures. Please keep in mind that taking one step at a time can make these easier. We are all at our own level sexually, so go at a pace that works for you. To help you progress, there is a range of adventures in this chapter so you don't feel too vulnerable. Take some risks, and the rewards will be like the pot of gold at the end of a sexy rainbow.

Good Vibrations

Here's an adventure you can try tonight! Experiencing orgasm while looking deeply into your lover's eyes and introducing a toy can be a truly powerful experience, as Juanita discovered:

Carlos and I started experimenting more with different sex positions. We ordered a Hitachi Magic Wand vibrator by mail. One night we were going at it pretty hot and heavy. We were doing it doggy-style, which has become my new favorite position. We had been at it for a few minutes and Carlos whispered in my ear that he had something special for me. He brought the vibrator around in front of me, turned it on, and put it in my hand. His hand was on top of mine, and together we slowly lowered it to my clitoris. The vibration was very strong and almost took my breath away.

Carlos pulled out of me slowly from behind, and I put the toy down. He turned me around to face him and sat down on the bed with his legs out before him. He pulled me toward him so I was squatting down, and I slipped him back inside me. I wrapped my legs around his back and looked into his beautiful, dark eyes. We sat still like this, with him throbbing inside me and connecting with our hearts and our eyes. He reached over and picked up the vibrator and together we held it on my clitoris. My breathing became heavy and I rocked my pelvis back and forth.

Having him inside of me as I did this was intoxicating. I could feel the exquisite sensations spiraling out from my clit building and building. I felt like I was going up a mountain, higher and higher.

Carlos matched my panting breath for breath. He let go of the vibe and held me firmly with one hand around my waist and the other on my neck. My eyes were half-closed as I rose higher and higher toward heaven. I pumped and rocked my hips faster, and Carlos' grip grew tighter. Then I was at the peak of the mountain with every muscle in my body rigid and tense.

I opened my eyes wide and saw love and passion in his eyes in a way I'd never seen. I saw his complete acceptance of me as his only woman. I jumped and soared off the cliff. My fingers dug into Carlos's shoulder as I held on.

I was electrified. Both of his hands were on my head now as we stared deeply into each other's hearts and souls. The moment went on forever as the vibrator fell to the side. He picked it up, turned it off, and held me tightly.

I felt waves of emotion come up and out of me as I realized I had just had my first orgasm and was able to share it with the one man on the planet who loves me unconditionally. It felt miraculous.

Grab Him by Surprise

Create juicy memories for both of you by manually stirring your man's desire, flirting madly with him and then stimulating your lover through his clothes while waiting on a ferry, in traffic, or any kind of car backup. If you're really brave and you have the appropriate privacy, go down on him to catch him by surprise.

Passing the time this way is not only fun but also creates food for fantasy for years to come.

Some restaurants have long tablecloths on their tables that give you ample opportunity to rev him up again. You may find your inner teenager comes out to play while you stoke his lust over dinner. If side by side, caress his leg and squeeze his thigh. If across from him, try playing your foot along the front of his pants to make him squirm in his seat. It's a very brave woman who quietly crawls under a table to find what she dropped from her purse. . . .

Dare to Find a New Rhythm

Surprise yourself by signing up for a class you normally wouldn't take. Local community centers often provide reasonably priced Latin or belly dancing classes. A new craze is hooping classes, using a hula hoop. These are tons of fun and a great workout. Get those endorphins flowing and have a quickie sex workout afterward, if you're so inclined.

For a more extravagant option, try a pole dance or lap dance class. These might be a bit harder to find, but even my local recreation center offers these classes. You may have to hunt a bit or travel to another town, and they may cost a bit more than regular dance classes, but they are worth it! They seem to feed directly into a woman's self-confidence. I have taken both and highly recommend them for *all* women. Exploration of other aspects of your inner sensuality is easily done in classes such as these. Take a chance on yourself!

Do a House Swap

How about a sexy camping adventure indoors? Trade houses with a friend and arrange everything in advance to treat your honey to an inexpensive trip. It may be only next door, but variety of location can do wonders for romance. Set it up so your and your friend's kids are all at your place so it becomes a treat for them as well. You can offer to do the same for them.

If you or your friends aren't comfortable sharing beds, then bring over sleeping bags and a blow-up mattress, or use their floor or couch. Bring over some candles, a bottle of wine, some cheese, and a French baguette from the grocery store and you have a night designed for love.

Check Out an Erotic Resort

For the more adventurous of you, explore "adult only" erotic resorts such as Hedonism (www.hedonism.com), Desire (www.desireresorts.com), Caliente (www.calienteresorts.com), and Temptation Resorts (www.temptationresorts.com) for clothing-optional adult fun. These resorts cater to couples who want to explore "alternative lifestyles" or swinging. There are no displays of public sex, but there are private playrooms where couples may go to experiment with other couples. This is a luxurious option offered at first-class resorts and one that may not be in your budget currently, but would be well worth saving up for if it tickles your fancy. What an incredible honeymoon or anniversary trip idea!

If you mention that you heard of them through Kim Switnicki and *Great Sex for Hard Times*, the good folks at Caliente Resorts will offer you a special goodie when you arrive.

Invite Others to Join In

You don't have to travel to a resort, though, to change things up. Many couples are curious about fulfilling the common fantasy of a threesome. Here's a way you can "test the waters" without undue risk to your relationship. Find an exotic dance club offering lap dances and take your man on a hot date to the club. You may want to try this out of town instead of at a local club. Have a drink or two to get warmed up, and enjoy the dancers. When you're ready, pick out a girl together and have her give your man a lap dance. Yoko took Jim to a club like this:

> It was dark inside and a bit smoky, but the loud, pulsing music helped it feel sexy. We picked out a gorgeous Latina woman who was tall and very curvy to give Jim a lap dance. I found it quite titillating to watch her get Jim excited. She performed her magic, bumping and grinding all over him. After her song, we thanked her and then chatted about how we were feeling. I found it quite a turn-on to watch him with her. He found it a bit uncomfortable, which was surprising to both of us. We stayed to finish our drinks and then went home and made passionate love.
>
> Next time we're going to have her dance for me and see what that feels like for both of us. I don't think it will lead to a threesome in our future, but the image of her writhing all over my husband will keep me hot for a long time! I can see now that we'll make lots of our own adventures as we grow together.

The key to having this work for you is the communication afterward. Discuss your feelings honestly about what it was like to see another woman with your man. Were you jealous, or did it turn you on? If you go the next step and have her dance for you with him watching, how does it feel for him? Use these feelings as a guide to where you take things from there. Adding another body to your bedroom can create countless problems for some yet for others it seems to be the perfect solution to spicing things up. Communication and honesty are crucial.

●●● Kim's **QUICKIE TIP**

Women in their forties tend to experience more sexual wet dreams! Rest assured that having sex with another man in your dreams is not an indication of infidelity or even that you want to have an affair—enjoy the thrills in your dreams with no harm done.

Check Out a Nightclub

Another extreme adventure could include attending a "play" event at a local or regional nightclub. In larger cities there are groups who will provide "alternative" nights for people to let down their hair and maybe their inhibitions as well. An event such as this might be a fetish night or a leather-and-lace night or a swingers night. You are often required to wear fetish clothing (leather, PVC, collars, chains, lingerie) or kinkier attire than you would see at a regular nightclub. The people who hold these events are regular folk like you and me. They are simply providing a safe environment for people to have fun exploring their sensual side in public. Boundaries are always respected for everyone.

These types of events are frequently, but not always, held at a local gay bar. These bars are fun to explore on any night for some great dancing and an atmosphere of respect and acceptance. You can safely expose more of your sexy side, usually without concern.

SEXY CHALLENGE
A Date for Love

You'll Need: Your and your man's schedules
Prep Time: 5 to 15 minutes
Cost: $0
Raciness Factor: Regular
Benefit: Improves communication

Schedule at least three dates for lovemaking surprises over the next three months and do it right now! Mark them in your date books, calendars, PDAs, or wherever you need to to make sure they happen. Some couples use secret symbols or codes on the family calendar so they are the only ones who know the dates for the love adventures. Other couples have the whole family participate in the scheduling so they all know this will be a date for Mom and Dad to be romantic.

* * *

Perhaps you aren't interested in expanding your horizons and simply want to create an element of suspense and surprise. Why not set up a scavenger hunt around your house or the neighborhood with sexy notes letting your sweetie know where to find the next clue on his way to his grand prize—you! Send him off to find items such as:

- Champagne glasses
- Sparkling juice
- Wine or champagne
- A corkscrew
- Massage oil
- A bottle of flavored lubricant
- A scarf or blindfold (let him know who will be wearing it)
- A sex toy (or batteries, just to keep him guessing)
- Matches (to light your fire or candles)
- A sponge to wash your back (if you are directing him to the tub)
- Whipped cream (to put on whatever body part he wishes—even one of his own!)
- Whatever else you can add to this list that will drive him crazy!

As I said earlier, each of us operates at a different sexual pace. But whatever your pace, the idea is to avoid getting into a rut. Perhaps it's time to create a "love jar," which can ensure an adventurous sex life. Develop a customized collection of romantic ideas, spicy encounters, nights of love, or even quickie ideas that are specific to you and your lover. You don't even need a jar. A special binder, a drawer, or even a shoe box will do. Use some sexy colored paper and pens to write out luscious, fun, and sexy ideas for the two of you to surprise each other with. Add to it whenever an idea comes to you, or after you read about one in a magazine or see one in a movie. This way, you can guarantee lust and desire—just grab something from the love jar!

Or consider expanding your personal sexual horizons by seeking out a fun sex-education class to spice things up. Check out local community colleges, universities, or love shops, or look online. I have a special treat to get you started. On the secret Web site page for readers of this book is a link for you to download an audio copy of my live G-spot workshop for free! Go to www.kimswitnicki.com/greatsexforhardtimes to download it. Pushing yourself to explore and learn new things is not only sexy but also proof of your commitment to keeping your love life exciting. Allow your risqué side to grow and shine and your love life will follow!

SEXY CHALLENGE
Switcheroo

You'll Need: A night out
Prep Time: 15 minutes to 1½ hours
Cost: $20+
Raciness Factor: Bold to Extreme
Benefit: Improves Communication

Switch roles and go out on the town pretending to be each other. Take it as far as you are able to while still keeping it exciting. Be daring and wear each other's clothes entirely, or be more discreet and perhaps only wear each other's underwear and coats. You may wear one of his ties or even a tie and shirt. He may wear your stockings under his pants. This challenge may depend on how close in size you are. Consider this option for Halloween if you want to feel "safer" while doing it.

Either way, go out behaving as the other would on a hot date. When you get home, spend at least thirty minutes doing to your partner what you would want them to do to you for a perfectly sensual experience. Enjoy the revelations!

We all need to commit to placing sufficient attention on our love lives, and there's no time like the present. If nothing you've read thus far sounds like something you can make happen *today*, then here's something you can do *right now*. . . . Book a date to play hooky with your honey. Pick a day or even an afternoon that you can both take off from work. What you do with those hours can be decided later, but at least for now you have set aside the time to be with each other. Remember to set this up by the end of this week, otherwise you'll put it off and may never do it!

chapter **18**

Erotica, Porn, and Naughty Letters— Engage All Your Senses for Electrifying Sex

Sex is a part of nature. I go along with nature. —**Marilyn Monroe,**

actress

Most men are more visual when it comes to sex, which means they prefer watching something to stimulate themselves (such as a video or pictures in a magazine) instead of listening to or reading about sexy situations. Most women are more auditory, so they can be aroused by listening to sexy scenes or romantic stories. However, I know lots of women who get very turned on by watching adult movies and lots of men who love to have sexy things whispered in their ears while lovemaking. There are no hard-and-fast rules, and all of us enjoy sexual stimulation more when each of our senses is engaged. Light some scented candles, have yummy treats available, and snuggle into each other with a naughty story or steamy film, or read each other a hot letter to spark some electrifying sex!

225

Erotica

Erotica (written erotic stories) is the number one sexual accessory around the world. The appeal of reading about others having sex is universal. Part of this may be because it seems somehow "safe" to explore your own hidden desires on the printed page without having to act them out. You can create the visual image in your mind and no one else can see it.

Erotica is a spectacular and simple way to discover more of what turns you on. Pick up a collection of erotic stories and you're sure to find that some turn you on more than others.

Typically, women may be turned off by language that is too strong or explicit. Men may prefer this more direct approach to naughty words, but this isn't always the case. Test the waters by reading some erotica and see if you like the dirtier versions or the tamer ones. There is no wrong way to enjoy it. Whatever turns you on and gets you feeling hot and sweaty is the ticket.

You can read erotic stories and poems written by people just like you on my Web site. I created a space for women to read erotica written by other women. Try your hand at penning a short, sexy story and submit it to me at www.kimswitnicki.com. I'll read it and may publish it on the Web site for others to share. Would your man be turned on by reading a hot story online that was written by you?

You can also write for yourself or for your lover's pleasure. When is the best time to write erotica? When either of you is leaving on a business trip or even just for the weekend, a short love note or an erotic story can keep the home fires burning. It doesn't have to be long. Grab a blank greeting card and write a line or two describing how you feel when you're in your lover's arms or what you want to do to him when he returns. I've even snuck into my man's suitcase before he heads out of town to tuck Post-its in his pants pockets. A simple phrase sent by e-mail or text can make your man's day too. These little spur-of-the-moment love notes can lead to some hot exchanges.

You can also write stories about fantasy characters if you're unsure how to write about you and your lover. Create fantasy roles and far-out scenes and read them out loud to your lover while he massages your back. Use lots of soft and sensuous words, such as words starting with the letter "s." You may feel more than his hands on you by the time you're finished!

● ● ● Kim's **QUICKIE TIP**

Any time you feel the urge, jot down sexy ideas or phrases and save them up for when you have more time to get your creative juices flowing into writing a whole story.

Practice writing an erotic letter to your man by doing some "free writing." First, daydream a little and imagine a hot scene with the two of you from an actual sexy encounter (or a fantasy scenario involving the two of you or perhaps others) and get a crystal-clear picture with as many details as possible. Then set a timer for five minutes and just start letting the words flow out of you as you describe what the people are doing and how they are feeling and try to use all of your senses to capture the small details. Tease the reader a little before getting to the main event and you're sure to have a winner. Start with a scene in your mind that gets you hot and simply describe the sensual images that you see. Have fun with it!

If you realize you're really good at writing erotica, you can make money doing it. There is a large market for erotic letters, novels, poetry, scripts for films, or even phone sex scripts. You can also write nonfiction erotica, such as sexy articles, movie cover copy, or movie or book reviews. What a great way to make some extra money!

SEXY CHALLENGE
Blinding Story

You'll Need: A scarf and an erotic story
Prep Time: As long as it takes to write or find some erotica
Cost: $0–$10
Raciness Factor: Bold
Benefit: Reduces inhibitions

Blindfold your lover (to help reduce both of your inhibitions) and read him an erotic story. The blindfold will enhance his other senses to take in the story in a more intense way. Give yourself bonus points if you write the story yourself!

Sexy Speak

Most women love to hear sweet nothings or naughty notions whispered in their ears. They love to listen to sexy stories and are often turned on by hearing their lover's (or their own) moans and breathing during lovemaking. You can purchase erotica on CD if you prefer listening over reading. At the time of this writing, the Web site www.awomansgoodnight.com provides the simple and sexy service of offering audio erotica for download and purchase. You can download erotic stories read by either a man or a woman. You can choose how explicit you want the story to be and you can even listen to a short clip before you buy. I recommend them if this appeals to you.

Visual Aids

Amateur video is becoming a popular hobby for a lot of couples. Now that we have digital video cameras and easy-to-use software, you can make a pretty fancy film of yourselves making love with special effects and a soundtrack! Marcia found out it can be a huge turn-on for people with regular and real bodies to see themselves making love on screen like movie stars:

> *Don and the kids and I took our annual trip up to my folks' cottage, which sits on a lovely lake with a small beach area. It's a tiny cottage, but with three separate bedrooms, hot and cold running water, and a small dock with a rowboat, it works great for a family holiday.*
>
> *We've been going up there for about ten years as a family, along with most of the other surrounding cottage owners. When Billy next door offered to take all three kids (along with his two) over to the fishing derby on the other side of the lake so we could have some private time, we jumped at the chance. They would stay for the barbecue and prizes and weren't expected back for at least ten hours. Whatever would we do with ourselves?*
>
> *Things in the romance department have been steadily improving since I opened up and shared how I wanted to spice things up for both of us. We spend more time together and it is intimate time where we really talk with each*

other. And I'm proud to say that since I opened up to Don, I haven't faked one orgasm! I don't envy other women anymore, because I can see how being vulnerable actually gets me more than I ever dreamed with this amazing man I married.

So here we were at this cottage, alone, with our video camera and sunlight streaming through the lace curtains in the living room. Now that Don knew how much lace turned me on, he had a new appreciation for the cottage décor. He was relaxed being away from work, and we had both spent the previous few days easing the stresses of life out of our bones. He came up behind me, handing me a cool glass of lemonade, and started rubbing my neck, his big, strong fingers melting any last pressures completely away.

I surprised myself a little by asking him if he wanted to set up the video camera so we could tape ourselves. His fingers hesitated for a minute on my neck. I kept my eyes closed, pretending that it was no big deal, even though my heart started to beat a little faster at the thought of us making our own porno! Then he resumed his massage, going a bit deeper and harder. I moaned a little, and he bent down and started kissing my neck. He worked his way up to my ear and whispered, "Wait right here." I sat down on the couch, which was right beside me. I watched him set up the camera on the tripod as I drank my lemonade. The condensation dripped off the bottom of the glass and down into my cleavage, startling me because my skin was so hot. My bikini top showed off the hardening of my nipples as the cold water dripped.

He watched me on the small video screen of the camera as he was framing the shot to keep the whole couch in focus. I decided to make it more interesting for him. I dipped my fingers in the glass, removing an ice cube. I put it to my lips and then moved it slowly down my chin, arching my head back as I slowly slid it along my neck and down toward my cleavage. I reached back with my other hand and undid my yellow bikini top. The red light came on the camera. I instantly felt myself get wet between my legs.

I proceeded to give him a show with the rapidly melting ice cube and my breasts. He soon came over to join me in our hot little movie. I found the video camera gave me a huge erotic push. It was like being watched, but in a safe way. I was a wild woman unleashed. Our sizzling adventure is stored on a tiny SD card that we labeled "Lemonade" and tucked safely away. It seems much safer than a videotape. We've only watched it twice, but both times it got us so hot, we never really finished watching the whole thing. We are both careful to put the card away after we watch our movie.

The kids didn't win any prizes at the fishing derby, but they had a blast. I felt like I had won an Oscar for my performance and look forward to the sequel.

Erotic movies are a powerful stimulus for the mind and the right one can do a wonderful job of turning you on quickly if you find it difficult to get turned on. They are also a wonderful prelude to warming things up for a date night.

Going into an adult movie store can be a fun and interesting experience. When you go in, ask the clerk for the couples section. Let them know you want a film with a plot, decent acting, and a director sensitive to couples. Anything by Candida Royalle is geared toward women. You can search online as well for couples movies. There are more quality films made now than ever before, due to adult films for couples gaining popularity.

Explore some mainstream movies with sizzling sex scenes first if the idea of adult movies is a bit too daring for you at this point. Some suggestions to get you started:

- *The Postman Always Rings Twice* (1946)
- *Barbarella* (1968)
- *Last Tango in Paris* (1972)
- *Body Heat* (1981)
- *Basic Instinct* (1992)
- *The Hunger* (1983)
- *9½ Weeks* (1986)
- *Two Moon Junction* (1988)
- *Henry and June* (1990)
- *Red Shoe Diaries* (1992)
- *The English Patient* (1996)
- *American Beauty* (1999)
- *Secretary* (2002)
- *Crash* (1996)

These films explore classic themes of sexuality, including lesbian sex, bondage, adultery, anal sex, and more.

Magazines are a good standard resource for erotic images, as well as for stories and letters. They are pretty easy to find and there are lots to choose from. Go to a store together and make it an adventure to select a magazine or two to bring home. What a wonderful surprise if you pick one out yourself to bring home to your man. *Playboy* and *Penthouse* have long been known for editorial excellence and fabulous articles. Really! *Penthouse* also has a *Penthouse Letters* magazine providing great erotic reading. Some magazines have classified sections in which you can find other couples or singles interested in swinging or other ways to get together for sexual exploration. Please play safe!

SEXY CHALLENGE
XXXtreme Shopping

You'll Need: A car
Prep Time: Enough to find an adult store
Cost: $0–$10
Raciness Factor: Bold
Benefit: Reduces Inhibitions

Find an adult store, either in your town or close by, and go with your lover and look around. Pick up any toys that interest you and look at them up close. Ask your man if any appeal to him. Wander around the shelves of movies and read the titles, look at the pictures, and pay attention to what tickles your fancy. They are usually set up in sections for gay, girl on girl, biracial, bigger women, older women, anal sex, large breasts, transvestites, transsexuals, orgies, and other categories as well. There should also be a couples section. If you can't find one, ask at the counter for a couples film and rent it!

chapter 19

XXXtreme Fun—Phone and Cybersex, Bondage, and Anal Play

Thou art to me a delicious torment. —**Ralph Waldo Emerson, author**

Warning: this chapter can take an ordinary sex life and make it sizzle and steam like cool water drops exploding on a hot skillet. If you are prepared to open yourself up to new worlds of possibility with spectacular results, hold on to your hat because the ride will be wild!

Take your loving to a racy, new level with cybersex. Turn up the heat with steamy phone sex. Let anal play breathe exciting new life into your bedroom. Break the bonds of boredom with some bondage and domination action. You've had a taste of these ideas throughout the book. Trust and mutual respect are crucial when exploring these more extreme roads to sexual pleasure. Now let's delve a little deeper into some XXXtreme fun!

Playing Safe

First and foremost, communication is key when playing with each other. I suggest you employ the use of "safe words" so you don't have to necessarily stop the "scene" that you are playing in. Try simple words such as "green," "yellow," and "red" to keep communication simple so your partner knows how far he can go with you. Come up with your own code if that is easier. You also want to maintain privacy so you both feel safe and comfortable and won't be interrupted while exploring new pleasure zones. Pushing your boundaries and your lover's can be like a pool of cool water on a hot day: refreshing and exhilarating. There are many books on the subject of BDSM (an acronym for different pairings and combinations of bondage and domination/discipline and sadism/sadomasochism/submission and masochism) if you wish to explore this avenue more deeply. Regardless of what the practice is called, remember that as long as you are both consenting and experiencing pleasure, it is all a part of healthy sexuality. Above all, have fun!

Anal Play

Anal play is best investigated when you are completely aroused so your body is more open and willing. You must be totally relaxed to receive anal penetration and, you may find that a gentle pushing out or slight bearing down makes penetration easier. Men and women both have two sphincters that must be passed through first, which may be uncomfortable at first, but after you get through them it is usually smooth sailing from there. Men often enjoy anal stimulation more than women (once they get over any phobias), since their prostate (the male G-spot) is usually best accessed anally. Women can still enjoy the feeling of fullness that anal penetration gives them, even though we don't have a prostate.

Toys for anal play are usually flared at the base or have handles so they won't get stuck or lost inside of you. Since the anus can be much tighter than the vagina, it is handy to have a handle to hang on to as well! The common butt plug comes in many sizes and provides a full feeling to the wearer when inserted. Anal beads are usually graduated in size, starting out small at one end and getting larger as you move up the line. I recommend only solid latex or silicone beads and not beads with string; the string poses a bacteria problem, since the string is too hard to clean properly. The beads are to be inserted (use lubricant) and then pulled out quickly at the moment of orgasm to intensify and extend the sensation. This can be a challenge with two of you, unless you are both clear who is pulling them out and what signal will be given when the right moment arrives.

Vibrating toys for anal use are usually smaller than regular vibrators and are designed with a graduated, flared base as well. Have double the fun if you are penetrated vaginally while having an anal vibrator in you at the same time. Your partner will be able to feel the vibration, since the rectum is very close to the vagina inside your pelvic floor.

Since we don't naturally lubricate anally, you must *always* use a lubricant for any anal play if there is to be insertion. Don't use "anal lube" if it has any numbing agents in it. This is unsafe, since pain is a signal that you should always listen to.

Ensure the anal area is clean and your nails are filed smooth and you have lots of slippery lubricant handy. Employ trust, relaxation, and solid communication, and you can open up a whole new avenue for lovemaking with anal play. Again, remember to have fun!

Domination

If the idea of experimenting with submission and domination makes you feel uncomfortable, don't do it. However, please note that the "rape fantasy," explained in chapter 11, is the most common fantasy for women. It does *not* mean you want to be violated, but rather that you want to be intensely desired by someone you are attracted to and want to give up control completely. The idea of being overpowered by someone you desire who also wants you with a ravenous hunger is incredibly appealing to most of us. Men included. As long as you consent to this play and the ground rules are established (keep it fun and playful), then it's all perfectly normal, acceptable, and healthy!

Spanking, pinching, biting, and other forms of intense sensation or pain during love play can be a confusing combination for people to understand. For others it may be a necessary part of the experience for them to achieve their peak of pleasure. We won't cover the intricacies of this area of sexuality but let's look at some basics.

First, as we become aroused, our pain tolerance is greatly enhanced so we can handle sensations we wouldn't normally be able to. As our excitement increases, so too does our ability to handle intense sensations. Plus, once you get in the mood, you are more present in your body and you can feel the sensations more. Men are usually able to get into their bodies much more quickly then women.

If you lightly run your nails along your forearm right now in a sensuous way and you aren't in the mood for romance, you won't feel much more than perhaps annoyance. If you were to read, watch, or think about something erotic and get slightly turned on, that same light nail-scratching of your arm would start to feel more sensual. Your senses would be attuned to it and you would be more responsive. If you were in the throes of passion, that same scratching may be barely felt at all. You might want a stronger scratching or pinching to achieve a pleasing result. Once you are on your way to orgasm, a more intense digging in of nails or light biting may be perfect. The same nail digging and biting while not turned on would be irritating to most of us.

The key to playing with more intense sensations or even a bit of pain is to start slowly and match the sensation with the level of arousal. This can take some practice, and communication is crucial! It's totally fine to say, "Ouch," or, "A bit softer," or, "Too hard, sweetie." You can also use code words (make up ones that work for you) such as "yellow" and "red" for "slow down" or "stop." Escalate the sensations to match levels of erotic intensity and see where it takes you.

Alison decided to be bold and brazen and went all-out for her and Bill's anniversary:

> *Bill got ready for work as usual on the morning of our twelfth anniversary. I had taken the day off because I had plans for us later to make the night memorable. It was a luxury for me to have a relaxing breakfast without rushing off to the office. Bill came to me for his kiss good-bye as I was cutting up some grapefruit for my breakfast. As he bent forward to brush his lips to mine, I grabbed the back of his head so we kissed hard. I remember how he had enjoyed my aggression, holding his arms above his head over by the fridge, on a previous encounter. I pulled away and whispered in his ear, "Tonight I'm going to make you moan, groan, and whimper like a little boy." And then I suckled his neck like a vampire, gently using my teeth. He let out a tiny moan and held me tightly. I slapped his bottom and shooed him out the door. I smiled when I saw the look of bewilderment on his face.*

I called him before lunchtime on his private office landline, since what I had to say was too private for a cell phone and because of potential snooping. I told him to go to the bathroom and remove his underwear so he was commando all day. I shared how I was lying on the bed naked, playing with myself with my free hand as I imagined him walking around that big office with all those people who didn't know he wasn't wearing underwear and how hot it was getting me. I slipped my finger into myself and then brought it up to my mouth, making slurping sounds so he could hear. I told him to shower at the office before coming home and make sure his bottom was squeaky clean—every inch of it, because I had something special planned for him. Click. I hung up before he could speak.

I made two other similar calls that day. One was to tell him, "Be home at precisely six o'clock and not a minute sooner or later or you will be punished." The other was to let him hear me orgasm as I made myself come over the phone while he listened. It was so hot! I was having a great time being the leader and imagining him squirming with a hard-on all day.

When he got home (at precisely six o'clock) I greeted him wearing stockings, a garter belt, my favorite black and red corset, and a huge naughty grin. I was holding a long red scarf in one hand and a bottle of our favorite flavored lubricant in the other. He dropped his briefcase and practically ran to me. He whispered, "I've been hard all day and can't wait to sink myself deep into you." I was melting in his arms and had to make an effort to stay standing and continue my role as woman in charge.

I explained that I had a game for us to play and it involved some pushing of both of our limits and asked if he was willing to play with me. We agreed on the ground rule of having "safe words." We decided on "red" for stopping the activity, "yellow" for caution that it was time to slow down, and "green" for full steam ahead. Not overly creative, but clear enough for us to both feel comfortable.

I wrapped the scarf around his eyes and led him to the living room, where I had a big, fluffy blanket laid out on the floor, lots of pillows, drinks and nibbles, and some toys, and the aroma of the vanilla-scented candles was starting to fill the room. I undressed him, laid him down, and fed him some of the fruit I had cut up earlier. In between bites I put a clothespin on each of his nipples, squeezing gently and listening to his moan of pleasure. I used another scarf to tie his hands above his head, checking in with him that this was okay. His erection stood straight up.

I had picked up some body wax at a love boutique earlier that week. The clerk explained that it had a lower melting point than regular wax and that I could even use it to massage my lover once it was melted. What a brilliant invention! I spent a half hour melting and dripping the wax all over Bill's body, alternating the warmth of it with the cooling of a rapidly melting ice cube from a cup I had ready. I would build the tension until he made a whimpering sound and would then stop so I didn't get to the "yellow" or "red" word. Then I would rub the wax into his skin and feel him relax until I dribbled more wax onto him. He started to groan with his need for release, but I wasn't done yet.

I rolled him onto his stomach and then brought him up so he was on his hands and knees with his bound hands in front of him. I whispered in his ear how much I loved him as I started massaging his beautiful butt. I had explored anal play with other lovers, but never with Bill, because he didn't want to. Now it seemed he was open and prepared for anything.

I generously lubed up his anus and the tiny anal toy I had purchased. I had learned I had to go slowly and gently because there were two different spots to pass through. I eased the toy in little by little and soon realized he was pushing back to help me slide the toy in farther. I was so turned on knowing I was penetrating my husband. It was intensely erotic. Once the toy was in deep and past the two sphincters, I started to slowly pull it out and push it in while he rocked back and forth with me. My free hand was still covered with lube, so I reached under him and grabbed his penis, which was rock hard. I squeezed it and he made a guttural sound I'd never heard before. I started to stroke his penis and he started bucking and pushing back into the toy and I thought I was going to climax right there. The bucking got faster, then he made a loud groan and the bucking stopped suddenly (as did my hands), and he squirted all over the fluffy blanket, shooting almost up to where his head was!

It was so intense, I let go of him and the small butt plug (which remained inside him) and dropped myself down onto my back with my face under his. He leaned forward and kissed me hungrily. I knew we had crossed a threshold, and this was only the beginning.

Bondage

One of the greatest inhibition-busters available is a blindfold. Whether on you or your lover, it helps you surrender to the power of the moment. Other senses are enhanced when your eyes are hidden and you can slip into fantasy and other personas much more easily. Bring your inner sensuality closer to the surface and out to play!

There are bondage items you can purchase online or in adult specialty stores, but you likely already have lots of sexy equipment around your house to experiment with first. As Alison discovered, clothes pins, ice cubes, and a scarf are simple tools for sexy, bold fun. You can also use elastics for tying around nipples or wrists, feathers for teasing while bound, a hairbrush for soft spanking or running along aroused skin, a soft rope for more exotic knot play (Japanese rope tying is an art form to some), or a bottle scrubber for tingly skin sensations. What other items can you think of for delicious torturing and teasing of your lover?

SEXY CHALLENGE
Tie Me Up, Tie Me Down!

You'll Need: Stockings, ability to tie a slipknot
Prep Time: None
Cost: $0
Raciness Factor: Extreme
Benefit: Improves Sexual Skills

Tie your man to a chair with your stockings using a slipknot (so he can reach down with his teeth to untie himself), and tease and pleasure him for a full hour before letting him have his release. Use all of the techniques you have learned in this book to rock his world, so he realizes that you truly are his sexual fantasy come alive!

Phone Sex

Phone sex involves talking sexy over the phone and masturbating. One or both (or all) parties may be doing the talking and/or masturbating. You can pay for this "service" using a commercial phone number, either receiving a recorded message or talking with a live person (or a group party line) on the other end. This can be a useful option as a first step to help you become more confident in your sexy-talk skills.

Lots of us dive right in to sexy phone talk because we find that being on the phone helps us be less inhibited, and dirty talk can be much easier when you can't see your lover. Make sure you're in a private and comfortable place and take the time to get relaxed or aroused before you get on the phone so you are prepared to get right to it. This is wildly successful as a method for long-distance lovers to stay connected. The use of cell phones has increased phone sex due to the flexibility of where you can go with your phone. It sure would make sitting in rush-hour traffic more exciting!

Engaging Technology

Cybersex is using instant messaging or another chat service—e-mail, chat rooms, webcams, or other Internet-based services—to engage your partner in sex talk while one or both of you masturbates. All you need are two computers (or even a Black-Berry or iPhone) to connect with each other. You don't need to be at different locations. I know of one couple who routinely sends erotic messages to each other, even when they are both at home but in separate parts of the house! It doesn't always lead to masturbation, but is great foreplay. When my honey and I are apart from each other, our BlackBerrys become great sex toys, keeping us erotically connected. You can incorporate sending pictures or short videos of yourselves to really steam things up. Just be aware that they are crossing cyberspace and may get into the wrong hands, so don't send anything you wouldn't want to potentially go public!

Try your hand at texting, sexting (sending erotic photos), or e-mailing a small sexy message and have your partner add on and reply so it keeps getting hotter and hotter. This is especially fun if one of you is on the way home to the other—great foreplay twenty or thirty minutes before connecting in the flesh! Here are some suggested intros to test the waters:

- "What are you wearing?"
- "Do you know what I was just doing?"
- "I had a hot, sexy dream last night. . . ."
- "I'm about to get into the shower."
- "I just got out of the shower."
- "I'm imagining what I'm going to do to you when you get here."
- "What would you like me to do to you when you get here?"

SEXY CHALLENGE
Backdoor, Please

You'll Need: Lubricant, anal beads (optional), blindfold (optional), latex glove (optional)
Prep Time: None
Symbols: $0
Raciness Factor: Extreme
Benefit: Improves Sexual Skills

Seduce your man in whatever way works best for you. First, ensure he is squeaky clean; maybe you can shower together first. Get him hot and horny, and eventually get him onto his hands and knees. You may blindfold him if you wish to help him release his inhibitions (and maybe yours, as well). Caress and make love to his bottom with your hands, your mouth, and your tongue, paying only occasional attention to his penis. Run your hands along his thighs and whisper in his ears how much you love his butt or his legs. Get him even hotter by rubbing your pubic area up against his legs so he can feel your moisture. Try slipping a finger or two into your vagina and then into his mouth so he can taste your juices.

Make sure you have the lubricant handy. After arousing him a good long while, slowly circle your finger or tongue around his anus so he gets comfortable with you in this super-sensitive area. Slowly slip the anal beads into him one by one, pausing after each to ensure he is comfortable. If he prefers a finger instead of the beads, wear a latex glove for the safest approach. Use lots of lubricant and slowly slip your finger in, letting him push back into you to guide you. Aim toward his tummy and you may soon feel his prostate (roughly walnut sized and shaped). Rubbing of the prostate may bring him to orgasm without touching his penis.

Pay attention to his signals whether you use the beads or your finger and have an amazing time!

chapter 20

Sexy Coupons, Games, and Notes to Get You Started— No More Excuses!

Women like me because I make them laugh. And what is an orgasm, except laughter of the loins? —**Mickey Rooney, actor**

What follows is a collection of ideas for fun, sexy games, and simple ways to get started having great sex if you aren't already! You'll also find some coupons that you can cut out or copy to give to your lover. No matter how tough times get or how hard things may seem, great sex is within your grasp. Reach out and grab it for all you're worth!

Sexiest To-Do List Ever!

There is a film called *The Bucket List*, starring Jack Nicholson and Morgan Freeman, about two old men who have terminal illnesses. They prepare lists of things to do before they "kick the bucket." Why not prepare a bucket list of all the sexual encounters you desire and want to attempt before it's too late? This can be an ongoing, fun exercise for stimulating your sensual creativity and keeping your sex life spontaneous and interesting. Once you have a draft, consider sharing and comparing lists with your man to see if there are any matching items you can tackle right away.

Feel free to decorate your list with a colored marker, a spritz of cologne, lipstick, sexy pictures, scrapbooking goodies, or anything else that turns you on.

Charm Your Lover with Sexy Wordplay

Entice your man with some sexy talk. Use the following phrases with your lover and challenge yourself to come up with some of your own.

> "When you _____ me, I just get so _____ that it makes me _____."
> "I'd love to take your _____ and _____ it until I (or you) _____."
> "Every time you _____ me, it makes me want to _____ you so much more."
> "Ohhh. That makes me so _____."

Creating an erotic story, one line at a time, with your partner can also be great fun and just the right prelude to a fabulous romp. You can start the story with "Once upon a time there was a beautiful woman whose only wish was to seduce her man, so this is how she started." Then see where he takes it and build on it back and forth. This is a great way to have some laughs and also to see just how far your lover is comfortable with sexy talk.

Sexy Games

As yet another bonus for you, if you go to the special Web page I created for readers of this sexy little book, you can download a copy of my Lioness Deluxe Sexy Feather Game, which I created to help people discover their erogenous zones. This game will help you learn how to communicate effectively, and you'll *really* get to know each other's bodies intimately. Take your time with the game, indulge each other, and prepare for an erotic adventure. Go to www.kimswitnicki.com/greatsexforhardtimes for your complimentary copy.

Rebecca Rosenblat, relationship and sexuality therapist, TV and radio host, and author of many wonderful sex books, offers this game for your pleasure:

> *Take any game—a board game, a card game, a sporting activity—and play it for forfeit. Just as strip poker requires forfeiting clothes, and pool can result in forfeiting money, you can change the rules so that the winner gets to have a sexual wish granted. For example, "Eight ball in the corner pocket and you get tied to the bed tonight." Or, "If I win at Monopoly, I get to have a sexual fantasy fulfilled by you." Or, "The winner at tennis gets to have the loser strip for them." You get the idea. This is a good starting point to open up discussions around role playing and whatever else you like.*

Another fun, enlightening game involves a "his and hers foreplay map," which can teach you more about how you engage in foreplay proceeding your lovemaking. On two single pieces of paper, each of you draws a stick person or other simple diagram of your own body. You each get a diagram of yourself and a diagram of your partner.

Then take the page with your own body image on it and note down on the drawing—in order, by number—the areas of your body that you like to have touched. Indicate back or front if it isn't obvious. For example, if you like to have your neck touched first, put a "1" by your neck. If you like to have your lips kissed, and then your breasts rubbed, you put a "2" on your lips and a "3" on your breasts. When done, take the page with your lover's body on it and note what areas you *think* your lover likes to have touched in order, by number.

When you are both complete, share the results and see how close you each came to matching what your partner truly wishes. It is quite likely that you will each end up adjusting your foreplay approach after this informative little game. How wonderful to learn something new in such a fun way!

Coupons

Here are some ideas for words to put on handmade or typed coupons to help get your creativity moving in fun, sexy ways:

- I invite you to share a body-to-body massage with no hands for ten minutes.
- I invite you to create an erotic story with me.
- I invite you for a relaxing foot rub with no talking—fantasizing only.
- I invite you into the shower so I can wash your, um, back.

- I invite you to watch me pleasure myself for your eyes only.
- I invite you to spend ten minutes mirroring me as I caress my body and we look into each other's eyes.
- I invite you for a candlelight dinner—clothing optional. All I'll be wearing is a smile and an apron as I serve it to you.
- I invite you for a quickie in the location of your choosing.
- I invite you to share three places on your body you want me to kiss you.
- I invite you to trade whispered fantasies with me.

💜 Have fun deepening your intimacy, communication, and chances for even better sex!

Sexy Notes

Remember, quickie invitations for love and romance can be delivered almost any time by e-mail, text, instant message, phone message, regular mail or courier, wrapped around a pet's collar, delivered by a friend, in lipstick on panties or on a mirror, on Post-it notes, in a lunch bag/briefcase/portfolio, on a rearview mirror, in a medicine cabinet, on or under a pillow, on or in a laptop, in a book, in his pants or jacket pocket, under a dinner plate or glass, on a hanger, and hundreds of other ways, so don't waste any opportunity to show him you care.

Get Lucky Note

If you wanna get lucky, try doing the _____ (fill in "laundry," "dishes," "ironing," "putting the kids to bed or bath," "pick up the groceries," etc.) and in exchange, because you are giving me the space and luxury of your big, strong shoulders to help with the load, you will get _____ (either be specific or simply say, "some romance tonight when we hit the sheets" or "lucky in the laundry room."

Come Meet Me Note

I see three qualities in you that are unique, and that deepens my love for you each day. I love that you are/have _____ , _____ and _____. Meet me at _____ so that I can _____.

Special Dessert Note

Dinner will be ready at _____ and you will have thirty minutes afterward to shower, relax, and prepare yourself for an amazing evening. First I will _____ and then you can expect _____ and we can top it off with _____.

A Chocolate-Covered Treat Note

Enclosed is a piece of _____ (tuck in his favorite chocolate bar, candy, or other edible treat). I can't wait for you to come home and go to our room, where I'll be lying on the bed naked with the rest of the _____ nestled in special places for you to nibble on.

XOXO Note

My favorite place to kiss you is on your _____ be-cause it makes me feel _____ and it reminds me of

_____. If you want me to kiss this special place, then come find me. I'm waiting for you _____.

Let's Make a Playdate Note

The next time you play with yourself, I want you to imagine me _____ and I will think of you _____ the next time I play with myself. Shall we make a date to enjoy watching each other?

Delicious Phrases to Use with Your Lover

Though this is not much of a game, you will definitely score if you surprise your partner with one (or more) of the below phrases!

I've always wanted to try _____.

I love it especially when you _____.

The three places I love to be touched the most are _____, _____, and _____.

My favorite type of thrusting when we have intercourse is (slow, quick, deep, shallow, varied, side to side, etc.) _____.

When we kiss, I especially love _____ more than _____.

When it comes to sex positions, we could use less _____ and more _____.

I prefer it when you _____ more than when you _____.

When we use sex toys, I'd like it if we did more _____ and less _____.

The next time you perform oral sex on me, I'd love it if you

_____.

When it comes to initiating sex, I'd like _____.

●●● Kim's **QUICKIE TIP**

Keep in mind that lovely scents slow our breathing, keep us calm, and can set a mood. Vanilla, spices, pumpkin pie, and patchouli are essences men respond well to, and women respond to rose, licorice, cucumber, and jasmine scents. You can drop essential oils onto a diffuser or lightbulb in your room, or keep an open potpourri dish out where you can inhale the fragrance as you walk by. The aroma of onions or fresh-baked bread when you walk in the door will also calm you. Even if it doesn't arouse you, if you can lose the stresses of the day, you or he will be more open to romance.

SEXY CHALLENGE
Baby Steps, Now

You'll Need: Nothing
Prep Time: None
Cost: $0
Raciness Factor: Extreme (if you haven't done any yet)
Benefit: Increases Inner Sensuality and Reduces Inhibition

If you haven't done any of the Sexy Challenges, I personally challenge you to find a nice easy one and go do it *right now*! It only takes one small baby step at a time for any journey—great or small. So take a step now toward your future, no matter how hard times get.

💜 Great sex can be yours tonight!

chapter **21**

Keep the Momentum Going—
Coaching, Commitment, and
Communication

A successful marriage requires falling in love many times, and always with the same person. —Mignon McLaughlin, journalist and author

There are no Sex Police knocking on your door to make sure you meet your lovemaking quota. There isn't an obvious penalty for letting your love life slip through the cracks into Humdrumville or worse, Nonexistentland. You are the only one who can make sure you don't end up with a boring, withered-up, useless sex life. Don't let all of life's little details get in the way of you having the powerful, erotic sex life you and your partner deserve to have!

Look back at all the fun you've been having and remember how great it feels after trying each new thing. Remember:

○ Having great sex makes all of life's little annoyances seem much smaller.

- Great sex makes all of life's small pleasures seem so much sweeter.
- Once you have great sex, you'll want to have more and more of it.

You now have the tools and methods to have the gift of great sex in your life, no matter how tough times get. And now you should realize great sex will make those tough times much easier to handle, because you're calmer, you're nicer to be around, you feel physically better, you smile more, and your partner enjoys all of these benefits too! Your job now is to keep yourself in the satisfying and rewarding place of having great sex regularly. Have you come to life like Michelle, who shares how she has come a long way and now is much happier with herself and her marriage?

> *I'm still enjoying my sensual baths with my mint bath gel and I spend bath time thinking a lot more erotic thoughts than I ever have before. I feel like a well has opened up inside me. The sexual part of me I thought was withering up and dying has come back to life! I'm going to keep my stock of flavored lubricant topped up and will keep trying out new kissing techniques on my husband. He says I look ten years younger, and I've started walking to lose some more weight. I never thought that something as simple as sex would give me my life back. Dave doesn't know how close I was to walking out. And now he never needs to. I love him in a way I hadn't realized, and I love me—which is the most important love of all, I guess.*

It's amazing how everyday workloads can have the capacity to overwhelm you and keep you from loving yourself, your body, and your sexuality, and from appreciating your partner. Resentment, bitterness, and irritability can easily build right along with tension. One of the ways we, as busy adults, can keep tension at bay is by making room for romance and not trying to do it all alone. Share the parenting and household commitment load. Remember to communicate with your partner and to let him know what it is that you need. Approach your partner from the "I need" place and not the "You have to/you should do" place. Once your partner realizes what he can contribute and the benefits of doing so for both of you, wonderful things will begin to happen, so you can both come together and enjoy more great sex!

Continue to develop your communication skills both in and out of the bedroom and you will not only deepen your sexual experiences, but you will also enhance all of your other relationships. Imagine how much easier your life will be when you become a better communicator. You also become an incredible role model for your kids. Revisit the communication chapter as often as you feel you need to. Improving communication is a lifelong event, so continue seeking ways, through either courses or books, to improve how you do it.

Be easy on yourself if your sexual plans don't go exactly as you had initially hoped. Things happen in life and sometimes we need to be patient, wondering when change will occur. There is a natural ebb and flow in all sexual relationships. My friend Dr. Trina Read, author of *Till Sex Do Us Part: Make Your Married Sex Irresistible*, explains this well in her book:

> *What is Sexual Rhythm? Sexual rhythm is a mind, body, spirit check-in to understand how much sex can be accommodated with your current life situation. Although sexual intercourse is important for your well-being as a couple, frequency is not necessarily the greatest common value. Rather, you aspire for maintaining a constant emotional and intimate connection.*

When you have little to no responsibility, your sexual rhythm can see you having sex often for hours at a time. Major changes or upheavals, like babies, promotions, or moving, mean sex will be irregular and an uphill battle to maintain any sort of regularity. When you aren't experiencing major changes and are gliding along without too many worries, sex on a weekly or at least on a regular basis is easily doable.

If you've been coasting along or painstakingly making sure to have sex once per week, it has likely created a negative reaction toward sex. When you understand your sexual rhythm, it puts you in the driver's seat, where you anticipate your current stage of life and make the necessary adjustments.

●●● Kim's **QUICKIE TIP**

Plan a regular check-in time, such as Sunday afternoons, to take the overall temperature of your sex life and see how you are both feeling about it.

Studies show the number one factor affecting your ability to make permanent change is having support. You have a variety of options available. Use this book to help enlist your partner for support so you both commit to placing time and attention on your love life on a regular basis. You can join forces with a friend who also wants to rev up her stalled romance engine so you can both urge each other to spend the time, commit to putting the attention on yourself and your man, and encourage each other when you slip up. Or you can engage the help of a sex coach, such as myself, for direct, focused, devoted time and attention on you and your relationship, you and your sexuality, and you and the great sex you deserve to be having each and every time!

The advantage of having a coach help you with your love life, instead of using your partner or a friend, is that a coach is solely there for you and has no other agenda or investment other than your pleasure and satisfaction. Women come to me when they have tried toys and read books but they still know there is something missing, something stuck or something blocking them from having the sex they crave and the relationship they deserve. They want an extra boost to their sensual relationship. They sometimes think they might need a sex therapist, because that is the only type of person they know of who can help people with sexual issues.

I'm here to say that if you think you might need sex therapy, consider that you may benefit from a sex coach instead. A coach helps you be accountable, stay committed, and actually take the time to focus on your sex life without letting everything else, including stress and frustration, get in the way. A good coach will help you sort out why you're frustrated, bored, or unsatisfied in the bedroom, and will offer you tools that help you sort out these issues quite quickly. Once you clear the clutter and find the answers, it becomes easy to create a positive upward spiral: *the more sex you have, the less stress you feel, and the less stress you feel, the happier you are, and the happier you are, the more sex you have. . . .*

Sex coaching is a collaborative relationship in which together we discover what your deep and true desires are, and then we lay out a step-by-step plan for you to get exactly what you need. We lay the groundwork, so you become supremely satisfied, not only each and every time you make love, but with your body, your self-identity, your sexuality, and who you are as a woman. You'll see how this empowers you in every aspect of your life, from your day-to-day encounters with shop owners, clerks, and people on the phone, to coworkers, friends, parents, your children, other family members, church associates, and, of course, your partner.

It can be difficult to make some of these changes without someone skilled guiding you in the right direction. If you find that you keep trying, but you aren't getting the results you need, crave, and deserve, call me to set up a private phone consultation, and we'll see if coaching is a good fit for you.

Success Bonuses

You can go to the special page on my Web site that I've set up just for you with links to the various products and resources I have mentioned in this book to help you in your quest for great sex. Go to www.kimswitnicki.com/greatsexforhardtimes to take some next steps for yourself. Here you can sign up for a free report on the "Top 10 Ways to Be a Sexier, More Confident Woman," subscribe to my newsletter—with tips on how to be a better lover and how to get more from your love life—read free erotic stories, sign up for courses, find out more about coaching, get information on live events, and more. You can also shop safely and securely for products hand-selected and approved by me for improving your love life. You can even listen to short audio lessons for ways to use some of the sex toys in my online shop! Be sure to check out my blog, which contains free articles on such fun topics as sexual anatomy, G-spots, orgasms, relationships, romance, sex ed, sexual health, sexy toys, and more. You can e-mail me at kim@kimswitnicki.com, join me on Facebook by searching for Kim Switnicki, or follow me on Twitter at Twitter.com/KimSwitnicki.

Something you tried in the past may not have worked well then, but now may be the perfect time to dust it off and try it on again. If a significant amount of time has passed, or if you have tried some of the fun challenges in this book, your confidence and comfort—and even your skill—may be much more developed at this time, so take a chance and try some of the things that didn't quite turn out as you had hoped in the past. They may be a perfect fit for you now.

Commit yourself to take the time for lovemaking and you will *never* regret it. You can have countless days and nights of sensual experiences, love-drenched orgasms, and powerful intimacy that your friends will envy. All you need to do is take one step at a time and keep going.

SEXY CHALLENGE
Commit to Us

You'll Need: A date book or other scheduling device
Prep Time: 15+ minutes
Cost: $0
Raciness Factor: Regular
Benefit: Improves Communication

Make a commitment in your date book, personal digital assistant, BlackBerry, or calendar (even get your assistant or kids on board) to have a "date" and pick a page or chapter from this book to use to stimulate your creativity. Pick one day per month for six months and also make a note to schedule more—and reward yourself for doing it!

●●○ Kim's **QUICKIE TIP**

Consider using the evening before each holiday as a hot date, since it is easy to remember, and you can likely sleep in afterward!

SEXY CHALLENGE
Challenge Diary

You'll Need: Paper or a journal, a writing instrument, sensual decorations (for the paper or journal)
Prep Time: 10+ minutes
Cost: $0+
Raciness Factor: Bold
Benefit: Increases Inner Sensuality

Set up a way to track when you do your Sexy Challenges—your partner *and* your sex life will love you for it. Decorate a journal or a few pages of paper with sensual images (a challenge on its own) to express your erotic-adventure spirit. Here are some ideas of what to write about for each challenge, to deepen the experience:

- "The most wonderful thing that happened was . . ."
- "We would modify this for the next time . . ." (such as items or accessories to be changed or added, prep time modified, location, time allowed for, etc.)
- "We discovered this about each other . . ." (sexually, physically, spiritually, emotionally)
- "We celebrated completing the Sexy Challenge by . . ."

SEXY CHALLENGE
Sexy Reminder

You'll Need: Internet access, Adobe Reader (to read the report; a free program is available at www.adobe.com)

Prep Time: None
Cost: $0
Raciness Factor: Regular
Benefit: Increases Inner Sensuality

Go to my Web site and download a free report called "Top 10 Ways to Be a Sexier, More Confident Woman," which includes a complimentary newsletter subscription so you continue to be reminded to have great sex!

💜 Push your sexual envelope and expand your sexual horizons. Once you do, you will soar over extraordinary rainbows of pleasure, be awash in gushes of satisfaction, and swim in the swirling magic of the pot of erotic love at the end of that rainbow. And it keeps getting better from there!

IMAGE CREDITS